Infection and Malignancy in Rheumatic Diseases

Editors

KEVIN L. WINTHROP
LEONARD H. CALABRESE

RHEUMATIC DISEASE CLINICS OF NORTH AMERICA

www.rheumatic.theclinics.com

Consulting Editor
MICHAEL H. WEISMAN

February 2017 • Volume 43 • Number 1

ELSEVIER

1600 John F. Kennedy Boulevard • Suite 1800 • Philadelphia, Pennsylvania, 19103-2899
http://www.theclinics.com

RHEUMATIC DISEASE CLINICS OF NORTH AMERICA Volume 43, Number 1
February 2017 ISSN 0889-857X, ISBN 13: 978-0-323-49675-9

Editor: Lauren Boyle
Developmental Editor: Casey Potter

Rheumatic Disease Clinics of North America (ISSN 0889-857X) is published quarterly by Elsevier Inc., 360 Park Avenue South, New York, NY 10010-1710. Months of issue are February, May, August, and November. Business and editorial offices: 1600 John F. Kennedy Boulevard, Suite 1800, Philadelphia, PA 19103-2899. Periodicals postage paid at New York, NY and additional mailing offices. Subscription prices are USD 335.00 per year for US individuals, USD 659.00 per year for US institutions, USD 100.00 per year for US students and residents, USD 395.00 per year for Canadian individuals, USD 823.00 per year for Canadian institutions, USD 465.00 per year for international individuals, USD 823.00 per year for international institutions, and USD 230.00 per year for Canadian and foreign students/residents. To receive student/resident rate, orders must be accompanied by name of affiliated institution, date of term, and the *signature* of program/residency coordinator on institution letterhead. Orders will be billed at individual rate until proof of status received. Foreign air speed delivery is included in all *Clinics* subscription prices. All prices are subject to change without notice. **POSTMASTER:** Send address changes to *Rheumatic Disease Clinics of North America,* Elsevier Health Sciences Division, Subscription Customer Service, 3251 Riverport Lane, Maryland Heights, MO 63043. **Customer Service: 1-800-654-2452 (US and Canada). From outside of the US and Canada: 314-447-8871. Fax: 314-447-8029. For print support, e-mail: JournalsCustomerService-usa@elsevier.com. For online support, e-mail: JournalsOnline Support-usa@elsevier.com.**

Reprints. For copies of 100 or more of articles in this publication, please contact the Commercial Reprints Department, Elsevier Inc., 360 Park Avenue South, New York, New York, 10010-1710; Tel.: +1-212-633-3874, Fax: +1-212-633-3820, and E-mail: reprints@elsevier.com.

Rheumatic Disease Clinics of North America is covered in *MEDLINE/PubMed (Index Medicus), Current Contents/Clinical Medicine, Science Citation Index, ISI/BIOMED,* and *EMBASE/Excerpta Medica.*

Contributors

CONSULTING EDITOR

MICHAEL H. WEISMAN, MD
Cedars-Sinai Chair in Rheumatology, Professor of Medicine, Cedars-Sinai Medical Center, Distinguished Professor of Medicine, David Geffen School of Medicine at UCLA, Los Angeles, California

EDITORS

KEVIN L. WINTHROP, MD, MPH
Professor of Public Health, Associate Professor of Infectious Diseases and Ophthalmology, Center for Infectious Disease Studies, Oregon Health and Science University and Portland State University School of Public Health, Portland, Oregon

LEONARD H. CALABRESE, DO
Professor of Medicine, Cleveland Clinic Lerner College of Medicine, Case Western University; Vice Chairman, Department of Rheumatic and Immunological Diseases, R.J. Fasenmyer Center for Clinical Immunology, Theodore F. Classen DO Chair of Osteopathic Research and Education, Cleveland Clinic Foundation, Cleveland, Ohio

AUTHORS

JOHN W. BADDLEY, MD, MSPH
Division of Infectious Diseases, Professor, Department of Medicine, Birmingham VA Medical Center, University of Alabama at Birmingham and Medical Service, Birmingham, Alabama

CLIFTON O. BINGHAM III, MD
Associate Professor of Medicine, Division of Rheumatology, Johns Hopkins School of Medicine, Baltimore, Maryland

PAUL A. BRYANT, MD
Infectious Diseases Fellow, Division of Infectious Diseases, Department of Medicine, University of Alabama at Birmingham, Birmingham, Alabama

PATRICE CACOUB, MD
Professor, Sorbonne Universités, UPMC Université Paris 06, UMR 7211, Inflammation-Immunopathology-Biotherapy Department (DHU i2B); INSERM; CNRS; AP-HP, Groupe Hospitalier Pitié-Salpêtrière, Department of Internal Medicine and Clinical Immunology, Paris, France

CASSANDRA M. CALABRESE, DO
RJ Fasenmeyer Center for Clinical Immunology, Department of Rheumatic and Immunologic Diseases, Cleveland Clinic, Cleveland, Ohio

LEONARD H. CALABRESE, DO
Professor of Medicine, Cleveland Clinic Lerner College of Medicine, Case Western University; Vice Chairman, Department of Rheumatic and Immunological Diseases, R.J. Fasenmyer Center for Clinical Immunology, Theodore F. Classen DO Chair of Osteopathic Research and Education, Cleveland Clinic Foundation, Cleveland, Ohio

LAURA C. CAPPELLI, MD, MHS
Instructor of Medicine, Division of Rheumatology, Johns Hopkins School of Medicine, Baltimore, Maryland

ELIZA F. CHAKRAVARTY, MD, MS
Associate Member, Arthritis and Clinical Immunology, Oklahoma Medical Research Foundation, Oklahoma City, Oklahoma

STANLEY B. COHEN, MD
Clinical Professor, Department of Internal Medicine, University of Texas Southwestern Medical School; Co Director, Division of Rheumatology, Presbyterian Hospital; Co-Medical Director, Metroplex Clinical Research Center, Dallas, Texas

CLOÉ COMMARMOND, MD
Inflammation-Immunopathology-Biotherapy Department (DHU i2B), Sorbonne Universités, UPMC Université Paris 06, UMR 7211; INSERM, UMR_S 959; CNRS, FRE3632; Department of Internal Medicine and Clinical Immunology, AP-HP, Groupe Hospitalier Pitié-Salpêtrière, Paris, France

ANNE CLAIRE DESBOIS, MD
Inflammation-Immunopathology-Biotherapy Department (DHU i2B), Sorbonne Universités, UPMC Université Paris 06, UMR 7211; INSERM, UMR_S 959; CNRS, FRE3632; Department of Internal Medicine and Clinical Immunology, AP-HP, Groupe Hospitalier Pitié-Salpêtrière, Paris, France

MARCIA A. FRIEDMAN, MD
Department of Rheumatology, Oregon Health and Science University, Portland, Oregon

ELIZABETH KIRCHNER, MSN
Certified Nurse Practitioner, Department of Rheumatic and Immunologic Disease, Cleveland Clinic, Cleveland, Ohio

CHRISTOS KOUTSIANAS, MD
Joint Rheumatology Program, Clinical Immunology-Rheumatology Unit, 2nd Department of Medicine and Laboratory, Hippokration General Hospital, National and Kapodistrian University of Athens School of Medicine, Athens, Greece; Department of Rheumatology, The Dudley Group NHS Foundation Trust, Russells Hall Hospital, Dudley, West Midlands, United Kingdom

XAVIER MARIETTE, MD, PhD
Professor, INSERM U1184, Assistance Publique-Hôpitaux de Paris (AP-HP), Center of Research on Immunology of Viral and Autoimmune Diseases (IMVA), Université Paris-Sud; Department of Rheumatology, Hôpitaux Universitaires Paris-Sud, Hôpital Bicêtre, Le Kremlin Bicêtre, France

EAMONN S. MOLLOY, MD, MS, FRCPI
Department of Rheumatology, St Vincent's University Hospital, Dublin, Ireland

VICTORIA RUFFING, RN-BC, CCRP
Nurse Manager, Division of Rheumatology, Johns Hopkins Arthritis Center, Baltimore, Maryland

DAVID SADOUN, MD, PhD
Inflammation-Immunopathology-Biotherapy Department (DHU i2B), Sorbonne
Universités, UPMC Université Paris 06, UMR 7211; INSERM, UMR_S 959; CNRS,
FRE3632; Department of Internal Medicine and Clinical Immunology, AP-HP, Groupe
Hospitalier Pitié-Salpêtrière, Paris, France

RAPHAÈLE SEROR, MD, PhD
Professor, INSERM U1184, Assistance Publique-Hôpitaux de Paris (AP-HP), Center
of Research on Immunology of Viral and Autoimmune Diseases (IMVA), Université
Paris-Sud; Department of Rheumatology, Hôpitaux Universitaires Paris-Sud, Hôpital
Bicêtre, Le Kremlin Bicêtre, France

AMI A. SHAH, MD, MHS
Assistant Professor of Medicine, Division of Rheumatology, Johns Hopkins School of
Medicine, Baltimore, Maryland

PADMAPRIYA SIVARAMAN, MD
Consultant Rheumatologist, Rheumatology Associates; Clinical Professor, Department of
Internal Medicine, University of Texas Southwestern Medical School; Co Director,
Division of Rheumatology, Presbyterian Hospital; Co-Medical Director, Metroplex Clinical
Research Center, Dallas, Texas

KONSTANTINOS THOMAS, MD
Joint Rheumatology Program, Clinical Immunology-Rheumatology Unit, 2nd Department
of Medicine and Laboratory, Hippokration General Hospital, National and Kapodistrian
University of Athens School of Medicine, Athens, Greece

DIMITRIOS VASSILOPOULOS, MD
Associate Professor of Medicine-Rheumatology, Joint Rheumatology Program,
Clinical Immunology-Rheumatology Unit, 2nd Department of Medicine and Laboratory,
Hippokration General Hospital, National and Kapodistrian University of Athens School of
Medicine, Athens, Greece

KEVIN L. WINTHROP, MD, MPH
Professor of Public Health, Associate Professor of Infectious Diseases and Ophthalmology,
Center for Infectious Disease Studies, Oregon Health and Science University and Portland
State University School of Public Health, Portland, Oregon

Contents

> Patients with rheumatoid arthritis are highly vulnerable to infections because of abnormalities in their immune system, and because of immunosuppressive effects of their medications. Vaccinations in this population are complicated by disease-modifying antirheumatic drugs, which also modulate or suppress the immune system and potentially decrease the immunogenicity and efficacy of the vaccines. We review the available data regarding the impact of rheumatoid arthritis therapy on the immunogenicity of various common vaccines. We also review rheumatoid arthritis–specific vaccination recommendations, live vaccine safety concerns, and current gaps in our understanding of these issues."

> For as long as there have been immunizations, there have been barriers to them. Immunization rates in the United States are below target. Rheumatologists and rheumatology practitioners need to understand the issues of immunizations in patients with autoimmune inflammatory disease to identify and overcome barriers to immunization. Several strategies for overcoming these barriers are discussed.

> Patients being treated with biological therapies are at increased risk for serious infections, including opportunistic infections. Although more is known about opportunistic infection risk with older biologics, such as antitumor necrosis factor drugs, there is less knowledge of opportunistic infection risk with newer biological therapies. The incidence of certain opportunistic infections (tuberculosis, herpes zoster, pneumocystosis) has been rigorously evaluated in large observational studies. However, data are more limited for other infections (histoplasmosis, nontuberculous mycobacteria). Infectious morbidity and mortality may be preventable with screening and prophylaxis in select populations.

diseases. Increased awareness of PML among rheumatologists is required, as earlier diagnosis and restoration of immune function may improve the otherwise grim prognosis associated with PML.

Herpes zoster is the reactivation of latent varicella zoster virus usually occurring decades after initial exposure, and manifesting as a painful vesicular rash occurring along one or more dermatomes. Zoster incidence increases with age as cell mediated immunity against latent virus wanes. Epidemiological evidence suggests that individuals with underlying rheumatic diseases are at increased risk for zoster. It remains unclear whether this is due to immunosuppressive medications or from immune dysregulation of the underlying disease. A vaccine against zoster is available for individuals 50 years and older. Theoretical risks remain about using this live-attenuated virus vaccine in immunosuppressed individuals.

Chronic hepatitis C virus (HCV) infection is associated with liver and extrahepatic complications, including B-cell lymphoma, cardiovascular and kidney diseases, glucose metabolism impairment and rheumatic conditions ie, arthralgia, myalgia, cryoglobulinemia vasculitis, sicca syndrome and the production of autoantibodies. The treatment has long been based on interferon alpha (IFN) that was found poorly effective, and contraindicated in many autoimmune/inflammatory disorders because of possible exacerbation of rheumatic disorders. The recent emergence of new oral IFN-free combinations offers an opportunity for HCV infected patients with autoimmune/inflammatory disorders to be cured with a short treatment duration and low risk of side effects.

Hepatitis B virus (HBV) reactivation (HBVr) has been an increasingly recognized and appreciated risk of immunosuppressive therapies in rheumatic patients. Despite its potential for significant morbidity and mortality, HBVr is a fully preventable complication with appropriate pretreatment screening and close monitoring of susceptible patients. Better knowledge of the risk for HBVr with the different antirheumatic agents and the establishment of the new-generation oral antivirals in clinical practice has greatly improved the design of screening and therapeutic algorithms. In this review, all available data regarding HBVr in rheumatic patients are critically presented and a screening and therapeutic algorithm is proposed.

RHEUMATIC DISEASE CLINICS OF NORTH AMERICA

ISSUE OF RELATED INTEREST

Medical Clinics of North America, January 2016 (Vol. 100, No. 1)
Managing Chronic Pain
Charles E. Argoff, *Editor*

Foreword

Infection and Malignancy in Rheumatic Diseases

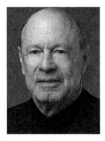

Michael H. Weisman, MD
Consulting Editor

This issue, edited and crafted by Winthrop and Calabrese, is spectacular. No one could have done a better job. The data and commentary will prove useful not only for what is state-of-the-art but also as a backdrop for research issues in years to come. Friedman and Winthrop discuss immunogenicity of vaccines related to the concomitant use of biologic agents—important issues are highlighted regarding the effectiveness of these vaccinations. They also address the gaps in our knowledge of the safety of live vaccines in our patients regardless of whether they are taking biologic drugs. Barriers to immunization are discussed in the context of public health and societal perspectives—an important contribution by Kirchner and Ruffing. Bryant and Baddley address the continuing problem of opportunistic infection risk with the use of biologic therapies and provide up-to-date information about the safety of different agents. The dilemma regarding malignancy risk is carefully analyzed by Seror and Mariette, noting the major contributions of both meta-analyses of clinical trials and essential information from real-world registries. We are generally reassured, as they indicate.

Bingham and colleagues provide new and timely information about the relationships among cancer chemotherapies and immune-related unwanted events—a potential new era of emerging rheumatic diseases brought on by advances in other fields. Sivaraman and Cohen address the management of RA and the risk of malignancies when utilizing Janus Kinase inhibition; this is clearly an emerging topic as the development of these drugs comes center stage. Calabrese and colleagues discuss progressive multifocal leukoencephalopathy or PML in the setting of our diseases and immune-suppressing drugs—the rare event causing a devastating outcome. Strategies to improve outcome are noted. Eliza Chakravarty provides a stunningly comprehensive review of herpes zoster incidence, pathogenesis, and prevention. The impact of hepatitis C and the rheumatologist is carefully analyzed by Cacoub and colleagues. The risk for hepatitis B reactivation during immunosuppression is continuing to be an ongoing problem for those of us that use biologic agents and care for rheumatic

Rheum Dis Clin N Am 43 (2017) xi–xii
http://dx.doi.org/10.1016/j.rdc.2016.10.002
0889-857X/17/© 2016 Published by Elsevier Inc.

rheumatic.theclinics.com

disease patients; Koutsianas and colleagues carefully talk about detection, prophy-laxis, and treatment.

I am notably and especially proud of this effort to bring so many important issues together in one issue in the *Rheumatic Disease Clinics of North America*. Congrats to the editors and contributors.

Michael H. Weisman, MD
Cedars-Sinai Chair in Rheumatology
Professor of Medicine
Cedars-Sinai Medical Center
Distinguished Professor of Medicine
David Geffen School of Medicine at UCLA
8700 Beverly Boulevard
Los Angeles, CA 90024, USA

E-mail address:
Michael.Weisman@cshs.org

Preface

Infection and Malignancy in Rheumatic Diseases

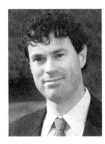 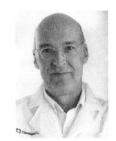

Kevin L. Winthrop, MD, MPH   Leonard H. Calabrese, DO
Editors

It is our pleasure to have worked with this outstanding group of authors in the production of this special *Rheumatic Disease Clinics of North America* issue on Infection and Malignancy in Rheumatic Diseases. This topic could be no more timely, as the pipeline of biologic and synthetic nonbiologic disease-modifying therapies continues to expand. With each new therapeutic, questions regarding infection and malignancy are revived. Only after many years of study, however, are the answers to such questions clearly elucidated. In this issue, top experts in the world bring us up-to-date in this regard. The articles herein highlight the risk of opportunistic and other infections in the setting of rheumatic disease. More importantly, prevention and screening strategies are reviewed and communicated in clinically relevant fashion with emphasis on latent viral diseases (eg, zoster, PML, hepatitis B virus) as well as vaccine-preventable infections. While time and years of study have largely ameliorated the fears of potential malignancy with Biologic therapy, important questions still remain. In addition, these questions have now resurfaced as JAK inhibitors and other small molecules begin to trickle into the therapeutic armamentarium. This issue updates the reader regarding the malignancy risk of these therapies, both known and unknown, and highlights the important areas of concern for the practicing rheumatologist. Last, Cappelli and colleagues cover the new frontier in rheumatology, highlighting new rheumatic syndromes caused by cancer immunotherapy.

Rheum Dis Clin N Am 43 (2017) xiii–xiv
http://dx.doi.org/10.1016/j.rdc.2016.10.001
0889-857X/17/© 2016 Published by Elsevier Inc.

rheumatic.theclinics.com

We trust you will enjoy the issue and find it both clinically useful and academically challenging.
Cheers,

Kevin L. Winthrop, MD, MPH
Center for Infectious Disease Studies
OHSU-PSU School of Public Health
3181 Southwest Sam Jackson Park Road
Mail Code GH 104
Portland, OR 97239, USA

Leonard H. Calabrese, DO
Cleveland Clinic Lerner College of Medicine
Case Western University
Department of Rheumatic and Immunological Diseases
Cleveland Clinic Foundation
Cleveland Clinic
9500 Euclid Avenue
Cleveland, OH 44195, USA

E-mail addresses:
winthrop@ohsu.edu (K.L. Winthrop)
calabrl@ccf.org (L.H. Calabrese)

Vaccines and Disease-Modifying Antirheumatic Drugs

Practical Implications for the Rheumatologist

Marcia A. Friedman, MD[a],*, Kevin L. Winthrop, MD[b]

KEYWORDS

- Vaccine • Rheumatoid arthritis • DMARD • Biologic • Anti-TNF • Rituximab
- Immunogenicity • Efficacy

KEY POINTS

- Influenza vaccine immunogenicity is reduced by rituximab and possibly abatacept, but is not reduced by methotrexate, anti–tumor necrosis factor (TNF) therapy, tofacitinib, or tocilizumab.
- Pneumococcal vaccine immunogenicity is reduced by rituximab, tofacitinib, and methotrexate, but is not reduced by anti-TNF therapy or tocilizumab.
- Live vaccines, such as shingles and yellow fever vaccines, are contraindicated in immunosuppressed patients, although observational data from patients inadvertently vaccinated while on biologic therapy suggest that this vaccine may be safer in the setting of some biologics than previously thought.
- Important gaps in our understanding include the efficacy of the newer 13-valent pneumococcal conjugate vaccine in the setting of rheumatoid arthritis, safety of shingles vaccine in the setting of biologics, and the impact of newer biologic drugs on vaccine immunogenicity.
- Rituximab profoundly reduces influenza and pneumococcal vaccine immunogenicity and vaccinations should be timed before rituximab or as long after rituximab dosing as compatible with vaccination schedules.

INTRODUCTION

Patients with rheumatoid arthritis (RA) are at greater risk of infectious complications, which is likely attributed both to medications used to treat RA, and to abnormalities in their immune systems.[1,2] Because of this, vaccinations against influenza, pneumococcus,

Disclosures: None (M.A. Friedman). Research support from Pfizer and Bristol-Myers Squibb, and consultant fees from AbbVie, UCB, Pfizer, Bristol-Myers Squibb, and Eli Lilly (K. Winthrop).
[a] Department of Rheumatology, Oregon Health and Science University, Mail Code OP09, 3181 Southwest Sam Jackson Park Road, Portland, OR 97239, USA; [b] Department of Infectious Diseases, Oregon Health and Science University, 840 SW Gaines Rd, Portland, OR 97239, USA
* Corresponding author.
E-mail address: friedmam@ohsu.edu

shingles, and other infections are important in the care of patients with RA. Unfortunately, vaccination rates for patients with RA in the United States remain low. Only approximately 28.5% of patients with RA in the United States are optimally vaccinated against pneumococcal pneumonia, 45.8% are optimally vaccinated against influenza, and as of 2012 only 4.0% of patients with rheumatic diseases older than 60 were vaccinated against shingles.[3,4]

As the arsenal of immuno-modulatory medications used to treat RA grows, important questions arise regarding the safety and efficacy of vaccinations in the setting of these medications. Safety of vaccinations has primarily been of concern with live vaccinations, such as shingles and yellow fever (YF), due to a concern of severe infections following live vaccination of an immunosuppressed patient on a biologic drug. As we discuss in this article, trials to evaluate the true risk of these vaccines in the setting of biologic use are not yet available, although observational studies of patients treated with biologics inadvertently vaccinated with live vaccines suggest they may be safer than previously thought.

Reduced efficacy of vaccines in the setting of disease-modifying antirheumatic drug (DMARD) use is a concern across all vaccination types. The efficacy of a vaccine in preventing an infection is difficult to measure in small trials, and typically these studies evaluate immunogenicity of a vaccine as a surrogate for efficacy. We currently have studies to evaluate the impact of a number of DMARDs on vaccine immunogenicity, which are discussed in this review; however, numerous gaps in our knowledge still exist and these gaps continue to grow as more biologic agents enter the market and vaccine formulations continue to change. In this review, we summarize the current available data for each DMARD and its influence on various vaccine immunogenicity. We also discuss vaccination recommendations and schedules as they apply to patients with RA, and summarize remaining gaps in our understanding of the influence of DMARDs on vaccine safety and immunogenicity.

RECOMMENDATIONS FOR VACCINATION IN PATIENTS WITH RHEUMATOID ARTHRITIS

Although all vaccines may be potentially important in patients with RA, in this review, we focus on influenza, pneumococcal, shingles, human papilloma virus (HPV), hepatitis B virus (HBV), and YF vaccines (**Table 1**). The first 3 of these are important for all patients with RA, whereas the latter 3 are relevant only in select patients. The influenza vaccine is available as an intramuscular vaccine and a live intranasal vaccine, the later of which is contraindicated in the setting of immunosuppression. The intramuscular vaccine is traditionally a trivalent vaccine protecting against 2 influenza A strains and 1 influenza B strain; however, recently a quadrivalent form became available that protects against an additional B strain.[5] All patients with RA should receive a yearly intramuscular influenza vaccine, and patients older than 65 should receive the high-dose vaccine, which has been shown to be more effective in this age group in the general population.[6–9] The high-dose vaccine is available only for the trivalent vaccine, and this high-dose vaccine has not yet been evaluated specifically in patients with RA.

The pneumococcal vaccine is available in the United States as a 13-valent conjugate vaccine (PCV-13), and a 23-valent polysaccharide vaccine (PPSV-23). Conjugate vaccines are generally more immunogenic than polysaccharide vaccines, although in patients with RA the previous 7-valent conjugate vaccine (PCV-7) was found to be no more immunogenic than the PPSV-23 vaccine.[10] The newer PCV-13 vaccine has not yet been extensively evaluated for immunogenicity in the setting of DMARD therapy, although 1 study so far has found lower yet adequate antibody levels in 22

Table 1
Important vaccines in RA and current recommendations for administration schedule

Infection	Vaccine Formulations Available in the United States	Indications for Patients with RA	Considerations Related to RA Therapy
Influenza	Intramuscular attenuated vaccine • Trivalent: 2 A and 1 B strain • Quadrivalent: 2 A and 2 B strains Intranasal live vaccine • Contraindicated in all patients with RA on immunosuppressive mediations	• Yearly vaccination in all patients with RA[6,7] • Patients older than 65 should receive the high-dose vaccine[a]	Rituximab: ideally give before start of therapy or as long after rituximab dosing as compatible with the influenza season.
Pneumococcus	PPSV-23: 23-valent polysaccharide vaccine PCV-13: 13-valent conjugate vaccine thought to be more immunogenic than polysaccharide[b]	• *All adults with RA should be vaccinated* • *Vaccine-naive patients*: PCV-13 followed by PPSV-23 ≥8 wk later. If younger than 65 at time of first dose, then repeat a single booster of PPSV-23 after 5 y. If first dose given after age 65, then patient does not need a further booster. All patients should be given one final dose of PPSV-23 after age 65 • *Previously vaccinated with PPSV-23*: Give PCV-13 ≥1 y after PPSV-23, continue PPSV-23 as above[12] • *Only 1 lifetime PCV-13 dose* • *PPSV-23 doses should be separated by ≥5 y*	When possible try to give pneumococcal vaccines before initiation of RA therapy.[7]
Herpes zoster or shingles	Live attenuated intramuscular vaccine	*ACR recommends shingles vaccine in immunocompetent patients with RA age 50 or older*[7,c]	• Contraindicated in all patients with RA on immunosuppression above CDC recommended thresholds.[d] • Contraindicated in the setting of biologics. • Optimal to vaccinate patients 4 wk before starting biologics or tofacitinib, or at least 1 month after discontinuation of such therapy (or longer based on the half-life of the biologic).

(continued on next page)

Table 1
(continued)

Infection	Vaccine Formulations Available in the United States	Indications for Patients with RA	Considerations Related to RA Therapy
Human papilloma virus (HPV)	Bivalent: approved only for female individuals Quadrivalent: strains 6,11,16, and 18 9-valent: above strains + 31, 33, 45, 52, 58	• All boys and girls at age 11 or 12 • Unvaccinated female individuals age 13–26 • Unvaccinated male individuals age 13–21, but extended to age 26 for immunocompromised men[18]	Vaccinate as appropriate regardless of immunosuppression.
Hepatitis B virus (HBV)	Single-antigen hepatitis B vaccine Combined vaccine with hepatitis A virus	Vaccination for all nonimmune adults who are at risk of HBV infection[e]	Screen for HBV before use of biologics, vaccinate if appropriate.[7,63–65]
Yellow Fever (YF)	Live attenuated intramuscular vaccine	Recommended for all immunocompetent adults who travel or live in endemic areas[17]	Contraindicated in the setting of immunosuppression.

Abbreviations: ACR, American College of Rheumatology; CDC, Centers for Disease Control and Prevention; RA, rheumatoid arthritis.

[a] High-dose vaccine is available only in the trivalent formulation, and has not been specifically studied in RA.[8,9]

[b] PCV-13 immunogenicity has not been adequately studied in RA. Studies of a prior conjugate vaccine PCV-7 was not shown to be more immunogenic than PPSV-23 in patients with RA.[10]

[c] CDC recommends 1-time vaccine in age 60+ within the general population due to cost-effectiveness and concerns for waning vaccine efficacy over time; however, this has not been evaluated specifically for patients with RA.[14]

[d] The CDC advises that the vaccine can be used safely with MTX (<0.4 mg/kg/wk, eg, 25 mg/wk); low to moderate doses of glucocorticoids (<20 mg/d prednisone or equivalent); intra-articular, bursal, or tendon corticosteroid injections, and azathioprine (<3.0 mg/kg/d); recommendation is based on expert opinion, minimal data exist regarding safe thresholds.[15,16]

[e] Nonimmune adults are those who are hepatitis B surface antigen negative. Risk factors include household contact or sexual partner who is hepatitis B surface antigen positive, more than 1 sexual partner in the past 6 months, those seeking evaluation for treatment of a sexually transmitted disease, men who have sex with men, current or recent intravenous drug users, resident or staff of a facility for the developmentally disabled, health care workers, patients with end-stage renal disease, travelers to endemic areas, patients with chronic liver disease, diabetic patients using glucometers, and patients with human immunodeficiency virus.[25]

patients with RA taking etanercept and methotrexate (MTX) compared with controls without RA.[11] For all immunosuppressed adults naive to pneumococcal vaccinations, the Centers for Disease Control and Prevention (CDC) recommends vaccination with PCV-13 followed by PPSV-23 ≥8 weeks to 1 year later. If patients have already received PPSV-23, PCV-13 should be given ≥1 year after PPSV-23. PCV-13 is a once in a lifetime vaccine. PPSV-23 given before the age of 65 is followed by a single booster after 5 years, and then a final dose after the age of 65; doses of PPSV-23 should be separated by at least 5 years.[12] This vaccination schedule, however, has not been specifically evaluated in the setting of patients with RA or DMARD therapy.

The herpes zoster or shingles vaccine is a live vaccine and is contraindicated in the setting of biologic therapy or high-dose corticosteroids. There are nonlive shingles vaccines in development that might eventually be a good option for this patient population; however, at this time only the live vaccine is commercially available in the United States.[13] This vaccine is approved for adults older than 50; however, citing differences in cost-effectiveness and concerns of decreased efficacy over time, the CDC recommends the vaccines only after the age of 60 in the general population.[14] These cost-effectiveness analyses were not done specifically for RA, however, and because of the high risk of shingles infection in these patients, the American College of Rheumatology (ACR) guidelines recommend vaccinating immunocompetent patients with RA who are older than 50.[7] Data are not available regarding safe levels of immunosuppressant medications at which the shingles vaccine can be given; however, based on expert opinion guidelines, the CDC advises that the shingles vaccine can be used safely with MTX (<0.4 mg/kg per week; eg, 25 mg/wk); low to moderate doses of glucocorticoids (<20 mg/d prednisone or equivalent); intra-articular, bursal, or tendon corticosteroid injections; and azathioprine (<3.0 mg/kg per day). If patients on biologic therapy are to be vaccinated for shingles, it is recommended to wait at least 1 month after discontinuation of biologics before giving the vaccine, or vaccinating 2 to 4 weeks before starting a biologic.[15,16] These wait times are recommended broadly for all immunosuppressant medications, but because the duration of immuno-modulatory effect varies greatly among biologics, this recommendation should be considered carefully in patients taking biologics with longer effect duration.

Several other vaccinations, such as YF, HPV, and HBV, become important for select patients with RA such as those living in or traveling to a YF-endemic country, those in a younger age group, and those at risk of HBV. The YF vaccine is a live vaccine and similarly to shingles is contraindicated in all patients on immunosuppression.[17]

The HPV vaccine is available as a bivalent, quadrivalent, and more a recently 9-valent vaccine; the 9-valent vaccine covers strains 6, 11, 16, 18, 31, 33, 45, 52, and 58, and is now the preferred vaccine. All male and female children should be vaccinated at age 11 or 12. Female patients who were not previously vaccinated should receive the vaccine between ages 13 and 26. Male patients typically are recommended to be vaccinated only through age 21; however, immunosuppressed men should be vaccinated through age 26.[18] The HPV vaccine should be given to any patient with RA if it would normally be indicated regardless of immunosuppression.[6,7]

HBV vaccination is of particular importance in patients with RA, as biologic therapy can increase the risk of reactivation in those infected.[19–24] Before initiating biologic therapy, HBV serology should be checked in all patients. Patients are considered to be immune if they have positive hepatitis B surface antibody (either by natural infection if they are hepatitis B core antibody positive, or by vaccination if they are hepatitis B core antibody negative). All those who are hepatitis B surface antibody negative are considered nonimmune, and vaccination is recommended for all nonimmune patients with RA with risk factors for acquiring HBV. Risk factors include having a household contact or sexual partner who is hepatitis B surface antigen (HBsAg) positive; having more than 1 sexual partner in the previous 6 months; seeking evaluation for treatment of a sexually transmitted disease; men who have sex with men; current or recent intravenous (IV) drug use; residing or working in a facility for the developmentally disabled; working in health care; traveling to endemic areas; having diabetes, human immunodeficiency virus, end-stage renal disease, or chronic liver disease; and using glucometers for diabetes.[25]

IMPACT OF DISEASE-MODIFYING ANTIRHEUMATIC DRUGS ON VACCINE IMMUNOGENICITY AND SAFETY
Nonbiologic Disease-Modifying Antirheumatic Drugs

Most nonbiologic DMARDs, excluding MTX, do not appear to have a significant impact on influenza vaccine immunogenicity.[26–29] MTX, however, does seem to adversely affect some vaccine humoral responses. Influenza vaccine immunogenicity is measured by hemagglutinin inhibitor (HI) titers, in which $\geq$1:40 is considered protective.[30] Studies evaluating the effect of MTX on influenza vaccine immunogenicity are somewhat contradictory, but overall suggest that although HI titers might be lower, most patients vaccinated while using MTX generally achieved titers adequate for protection against influenza infection.[26,29,31–33] MTX does, however, appear to reduce humoral response to pneumococcal vaccination, although only the PPSV-23 and PCV-7 vaccines have been evaluated in patients with RA on MTX.[32,34,35] MTX-treated patients vaccinated with these pneumococcal vaccines were less likely to achieve adequate humoral responses. A recent meta-analysis evaluating the effect of MTX on pneumococcal vaccine immunogenicity found decreased response rates to pneumococcal vaccinations among patients taking MTX compared with controls for both serotypes of pneumococcus evaluated (pooled odds ratio 0.33, 95% confidence interval [CI] 0.20–0.54, for serotype 6B; and 0.58, 95% CI 0.36–0.94, for serotype 23F).[32] Little is known about the effect of MTX on the immunogenicity or safety of the shingles vaccine. The CDC advises that the shingles vaccine can be safely given to patients with RA taking less than 0.4 mg/kg per week of MTX; however, this recommendation is solely based on expert opinion, as adequate data to assess this risk does not yet exist.[15]

Anti–Tumor Necrosis Factor Therapy

Most studies evaluating the impact of anti–tumor necrosis factor (TNF) therapy on influenza vaccine immunogenicity found that these patients generally achieve adequate HI titers for protection against influenza.[26,29,31–33,36–39] Anti-TNF therapy also does not appear to reduce humoral response to pneumococcal vaccinations.[11,31,32,34,35,39–41] The effect of TNF inhibitors of immunogenicity of the HPV vaccine has been evaluated in a small observational cohort of 9 patients with juvenile idiopathic arthritis, and found that all patients were seropositive after vaccination.[42] Two studies evaluating the immunogenicity of the HBV vaccine in the setting of anti-TNF therapy suggest that anti-TNF therapy impairs the humoral response to the HBV vaccine. One of these studies evaluated patients with inflammatory bowel disease (IBD) treated with either anti-TNF drugs or other immunosuppressants, and found that patients treated with anti-TNFs had a 46% vaccine response rate compared with 62% response rate in other patients with IBD not treated with TNF inhibitors.[43] Another study evaluating patients with ankylosing spondylitis treated with either nonsteroidal anti-inflammatory drugs or anti-TNF drugs, also found significantly decreased humoral responses to the HBV vaccine in those patients treated with the anti-TNF therapy.[44]

The shingles and the YF vaccines are both live vaccines and are contraindicated in the setting of biologic therapy due to concern of acquiring an infection from the vaccine in this setting.[15–17] To this date, however, no studies exist directly evaluating the safety or efficacy of live vaccines in the setting of biologic therapy. Observational studies looking at patients on biologics inadvertently vaccinated with live vaccines have not shown any infectious complications of these live vaccines, suggesting that live vaccines may be safer in this setting than previously thought. Two observational studies of persons inadvertently vaccinated for shingles while on biologic therapy (mostly anti-TNF drugs) found no cases of shingles or varicella in the 4 to 6 weeks of follow-up. The first study looked at claims data from a nationwide US health plan and found that of 47 patients exposed to biologics and given the shingles vaccine, none developed shingles or varicella in the 30-day follow-up time.[45] The second study looking at Medicare data found that of 633 patients on biologics inadvertently vaccinated for shingles, none developed shingles or varicella in the 6 weeks after vaccination.[4] Because patients with RA on immunosuppressive therapy are at high risk of developing shingles, studies evaluating the safety of this vaccine in the setting of anti-TNF therapy are necessary to improve the care of this vulnerable population.[46,47] The YF vaccine is also a live vaccine and is similarly contraindicated in patients on biologics. As with the shingles vaccine, no comparative studies exist directly evaluating its safety in the setting of biologics. During a recent outbreak of YF in Brazil, a number of patients who already had primary immunity to YF received booster YF vaccines while taking biologic therapy (primarily anti-TNF). In these patients, no cases of adverse reactions were found, and all were able to achieve adequate antibody titers; however, these data should not be extrapolated to those receiving the vaccine for the first time who would be at higher risk than patients being re-vaccinated.[48,49]

Rituximab

Of all RA therapies, rituximab has consistently been shown to have the most profound impact on vaccine immunogenicity. Influenza vaccinations are significantly less immunogenic when given to patients taking rituximab.[32,50–53] The timing of the vaccine in relationship to the rituximab dose also appears to be critically important, as vaccinations given 6 months or more after rituximab dosing have been shown to result in better humoral response than a short interval of 4 to 8 weeks.[51,52] Not surprisingly, rituximab also significantly impairs humoral response to the pneumococcal vaccines.[32,51,54,55] In a recent study evaluating the PCV-7 vaccine in the setting of rituximab therapy, only 10.3% of patients treated with rituximab monotherapy had an adequate response to both vaccine antigens evaluated. This effect was compounded by MTX use, in which no patients treated with both MTX and rituximab achieved adequate responses to both antigens.[54] No data exist regarding the effect of rituximab on HBV, HPV, or YF vaccines, although it seems likely that rituximab therapy would impair humoral responses to these vaccinations as well. Safety of live vaccination has also not been evaluated in the setting of rituximab therapy, and these vaccines are contraindicated in this setting.

Abatacept

Studies on vaccine immunogenicity in the setting of abatacept are limited. One study evaluating the impact of abatacept on the immunogenicity of the 2009 influenza A/H1N1 vaccine found significantly reduced humoral response, although newer trivalent and quadrivalent vaccines, which may be more immunogenic, have not been evaluated.[27,56] Abatacept also appeared to have a detrimental effect on humoral response to the PCV-7 vaccine; of 17 patients on abatacept being given PCV-7, only 3 achieved adequate responses to the 2 antigens evaluated.[54] Further studies are necessary to evaluate this question in the setting of currently available and potentially more immunogenic PPSV-23 and PCV-13 vaccines. Abatacept has also not been directly evaluated in the setting of shingles, HBV, HPV, or YF, and as with other biologics, live vaccines are contraindicated for patients on abatacept.

Tofacitinib

One study currently exists evaluating the immunogenicity of the 2011 to 2012 trivalent influenza vaccine and PPSV-23 and the in the setting of tofacitinib therapy. In the first part of this study, tofacitinib-naive patients were started on either tofacitinib or placebo and vaccinated 4 weeks later. Here investigators found that although both groups had similar proportions of protective influenza response titers, patients treated with tofacitinib had lower rates of protective pneumococcal titers compared with placebo (45.1% vs 68.4%). A second part of this study randomized patients already on tofacitinib to a group on continuous tofacitinib compared with a group undergoing a 2-week withdrawal period before vaccination to determine whether a drug-free period before vaccination would improve humoral response. Withdrawing the drug for 2 weeks did not result in any significant improvement in humoral response to either influenza or PPSV-23 vaccination. Tofacitinib has not been directly evaluated in the setting of any other vaccines.

Tocilizumab

In one trial of 111 patients with RA on tocilizumab with or without MTX compared with controls with RA, the antibody response to trivalent influenza vaccination did not appear to be any different between the tocilizumab-treated patients and controls with RA.[57] Patients with RA treated with tocilizumab also do not appear to have a significantly reduced humoral response to the PPSV-23 or PCV-7 vaccines.[54,58,59] One of these studies additionally evaluated the impact of tocilizumab on tetanus toxoid vaccine immunogenicity, and found no attenuation of humoral response to this vaccine either.[58] Further studies are needed to assess the impact of tocilizumab on HBV, HPV, YF, and other vaccines.

Prednisone

Prednisone use has not been shown to be a risk factor for reduced influenza vaccine humoral response.[26,36,60] Limited studies exist to evaluate the effect of prednisone therapy on pneumococcal vaccinations specifically in RA; however, a recent study evaluating the effect of $\geq$20 mg/d of prednisone on PPSV-23 immunogenicity in adults with a variety of inflammatory disorders found that patients treated with high doses of prednisone were less likely to achieve protective antibody titers.[61] Another group of 34 patients on prednisone (mean dose 7 mg/d, interquartile range 5–20) traveling to endemic areas were vaccinated for YF, 18 of whom were vaccine naive, and although these patients seemed to have an increased rate of local injection site reactions, there were no major adverse events and all patients demonstrated satisfactory immunogenicity.[62]

SUMMARY

Patients with RA are at high risk of infectious complications, and vaccinations are an important part of their preventive care. Unfortunately, a number of medications that are used to treat RA may impair the immunogenicity and efficacy of vaccines. Fortunately, the influenza vaccine seems to be reasonably immunogenic in the setting of most DMARD therapy, with the exception of rituximab and possibly abatacept. The pneumococcal vaccine immunogenicity studies have shown reduced humoral responses in the setting of MTX, rituximab, and tofacitinib, and therefore ideally would be given before the start of such therapy. HBV vaccines are likely less immunogenic in the setting of anti-TNF therapy, but have not been evaluated in the setting of other DMARDs, and the HPV vaccine immunogenicity also has not been directly evaluated in the setting of RA therapy. Both shingles and YF vaccines are currently contraindicated in the setting of biologic therapy; however, observational studies suggest they may be safer than previously thought, although this needs to be evaluated further with larger prospective trials.

Numerous gaps still exist in our understanding of vaccine immunogenicity and safety in the setting of DMARD therapy. Of particular importance are the newer PCV-13 vaccine, and the recommended pneumococcal immunization schedule, both of which need to be evaluated in patients with RA on various DMARDs to determine if this vaccine and schedule are optimally immunogenic for this population. The safety of live vaccinations in the setting of biologic therapy also requires urgent evaluation, as patients with RA are at high risk for shingles infection and commonly do not receive the vaccine due to their ongoing biologic therapy. It also remains unknown how most DMARDs affect the HPV and HBV vaccine immunogenicity.

Even though our understanding of DMARD therapy and vaccine immunogenicity is constantly growing, recommendations are often still dependent on poor-quality data or expert opinions to guide clinical practice. Furthermore, despite the importance of vaccinations for patients with RA, US vaccination rates remain quite low. In this review, we have summarized the available safety and immunogenicity data of vaccinations in the setting of DMARD therapy, and also have discussed gaps in our knowledge and important questions that still need to be answered. With more available information regarding optimal vaccine timing, and better data to address safety concerns, it is hopeful that rheumatologists and other providers will have better tools to guide clinical practice and minimize the risk of vaccine-preventable infections in this vulnerable patient population.

REFERENCES

1. Wolfe F, Mitchell DM, Sibley JT, et al. The mortality of rheumatoid arthritis. Arthritis Rheum 1994;37(4):481–94.
2. Glück T, Müller-Ladner U. Vaccination in patients with chronic rheumatic or autoimmune diseases. Clin Infect Dis 2008;46(9):1459–65.
3. Hmamouchi I, Winthrop K, Launay O, et al. Low rate of influenza and pneumococcal vaccine coverage in rheumatoid arthritis: data from the international COMORA cohort. Vaccine 2015;33(12):1446–52.
4. Zhang J, Xie F, Delzell E, et al. Association between vaccination for herpes zoster and risk of herpes zoster infection among older patients with selected immune-mediated diseases. JAMA 2012;308(1):43–9.
5. Grohskopf LA, Sokolow LZ, Olsen SJ, et al. Prevention and control of influenza with vaccines: recommendations of the advisory committee on immunization practices, United States, 2015-16 influenza season. MMWR Morb Mortal Wkly Rep 2015;64(30):818–25.
6. van Assen S, Agmon-Levin N, Elkayam O, et al. EULAR recommendations for vaccination in adult patients with autoimmune inflammatory rheumatic diseases. Ann Rheum Dis 2011;70(3):414–22.

7. Singh JA, Saag KG, Bridges SL, et al. 2015 American College of Rheumatology Guideline for the Treatment of Rheumatoid Arthritis. Arthritis Rheumatol 2016; 68(1):1–26.

8. DiazGranados CA, Dunning AJ, Kimmel M, et al. Efficacy of high-dose versus standard-dose influenza vaccine in older adults. N Engl J Med 2014;371(7): 635–45.

9. Izurieta HS, Thadani N, Shay DK, et al. Comparative effectiveness of high-dose versus standard-dose influenza vaccines in US residents aged 65 years and older from 2012 to 2013 using Medicare data: a retrospective cohort analysis. Lancet Infect Dis 2015;15(3):293–300.

10. Kapetanovic MC, Roseman C, Jönsson G, et al. Heptavalent pneumococcal conjugato vaccine elicits similar antibody response as standard 23-valent polysaccharide vaccine in adult patients with RA treated with immunomodulating drugs. Clin Rheumatol 2011;30(12):1555–61.

11. Rákóczi É, Perge B, Végh E, et al. Evaluation of the immunogenicity of the 13-valent conjugated pneumococcal vaccine in rheumatoid arthritis patients treated with etanercept. Joint Bone Spine 2016. [Epub ahead of print].

12. Kobayashi M, Bennett NM, Gierke R, et al. Intervals between PCV13 and PPSV23 vaccines: recommendations of the advisory committee on immunization practices (ACIP). MMWR Morb Mortal Wkly Rep 2015;64(34):944–7.

13. Lal H, Cunningham AL, Godeaux O, et al. Efficacy of an adjuvanted herpes zoster subunit vaccine in older adults. N Engl J Med 2015;372(22):2087–96.

14. Hales CM, Harpaz R, Ortega-Sanchez I, et al. Centers for Disease Control and Prevention (CDC). Update on recommendations for use of herpes zoster vaccine. MMWR Morb Mortal Wkly Rep 2014;63(33):729–31.

15. Harpaz R, Ortega-Sanchez IR, Seward JF, Advisory Committee on Immunization Practices (ACIP) Centers for Disease Control and Prevention (CDC). Prevention of herpes zoster: recommendations of the Advisory Committee on Immunization Practices (ACIP). MMWR Recomm Rep 2008;57(RR-5):1–30 [quiz: CE2–4].

16. Rubin LG, Levin MJ, Ljungman P, et al. 2013 IDSA clinical practice guideline for vaccination of the immunocompromised host. Clin Infect Dis 2014;58(3):309–18.

17. Staples JE, Gershman M, Fischer M. Centers for Disease Control and Prevention (CDC). Yellow fever vaccine: recommendations of the Advisory Committee on Immunization Practices (ACIP). MMWR Recomm Rep 2010;59(RR-7):1–27.

18. Petrosky E, Bocchini JA, Hariri S, et al. Use of 9-valent human papillomavirus (HPV) vaccine: updated HPV vaccination recommendations of the advisory committee on immunization practices. MMWR Morb Mortal Wkly Rep 2015;64(11): 300–4.

19. Nard FD, Todoerti M, Grosso V, et al. Risk of hepatitis B virus reactivation in rheumatoid arthritis patients undergoing biologic treatment: extending perspective from old to newer drugs. World J Hepatol 2015;7(3):344–61.

20. Ryu HH, Lee EY, Shin K, et al. Hepatitis B virus reactivation in rheumatoid arthritis and ankylosing spondylitis patients treated with anti-TNFα agents: a retrospective analysis of 49 cases. Clin Rheumatol 2012;31(6):931–6.

21. Mori S, Fujiyama S. Hepatitis B virus reactivation associated with antirheumatic therapy: risk and prophylaxis recommendations. World J Gastroenterol 2015; 21(36):10274–89.

22. Pérez-Alvarez R, Díaz-Lagares C, García-Hernández F, et al. Hepatitis B virus (HBV) reactivation in patients receiving tumor necrosis factor (TNF)-targeted therapy: analysis of 257 cases. Medicine (Baltimore) 2011;90(6):359–71.

23. Carroll MB, Forgione MA. Use of tumor necrosis factor alpha inhibitors in hepatitis B surface antigen-positive patients: a literature review and potential mechanisms of action. Clin Rheumatol 2010;29(9):1021–9.

24. Tan J, Zhou J, Zhao P, et al. Prospective study of HBV reactivation risk in rheumatoid arthritis patients who received conventional disease-modifying antirheumatic drugs. Clin Rheumatol 2012;31(8):1169–75.

25. Mast EE, Weinbaum CM, Fiore AE, et al. A comprehensive immunization strategy to eliminate transmission of hepatitis B virus infection in the United States: recommendations of the Advisory Committee on Immunization Practices (ACIP) Part II: immunization of adults. MMWR Recomm Rep 2006;55(RR-16):1–33 [quiz: CE1–4].

26. Fomin I, Caspi D, Levy V, et al. Vaccination against influenza in rheumatoid arthritis: the effect of disease modifying drugs, including TNF alpha blockers. Ann Rheum Dis 2006;65(2):191–4.

27. Adler S, Krivine A, Weix J, et al. Protective effect of A/H1N1 vaccination in immune-mediated disease–a prospectively controlled vaccination study. Rheumatology (Oxford) 2012;51(4):695–700.

28. França IL, Ribeiro AC, Aikawa NE, et al. TNF blockers show distinct patterns of immune response to the pandemic influenza A H1N1 vaccine in inflammatory arthritis patients. Rheumatology (Oxford) 2012;51(11):2091–8.

29. Gabay C, Bel M, Combescure C, et al. Impact of synthetic and biologic disease-modifying antirheumatic drugs on antibody responses to the AS03-adjuvanted pandemic influenza vaccine: a prospective, open-label, parallel-cohort, single-center study. Arthritis Rheum 2011;63(6):1486–96.

30. Couch RB, Atmar RL, Franco LM, et al. Antibody correlates and predictors of immunity to naturally occurring influenza in humans and the importance of antibody to the neuraminidase. J Infect Dis 2013;207(6):974–81.

31. Kivitz AJ, Schechtman J, Texter M, et al. Vaccine responses in patients with rheumatoid arthritis treated with certolizumab pegol: results from a single-blind randomized phase IV trial. J Rheumatol 2014;41(4):648–57.

32. Hua C, Barnetche T, Combe B, et al. Effect of methotrexate, anti-tumor necrosis factor α, and rituximab on the immune response to influenza and pneumococcal vaccines in patients with rheumatoid arthritis: a systematic review and meta-analysis. Arthritis Care Res (Hoboken) 2014;66(7):1016–26.

33. Kapetanovic MC, Saxne T, Nilsson JA, et al. Influenza vaccination as model for testing immune modulation induced by anti-TNF and methotrexate therapy in rheumatoid arthritis patients. Rheumatology (Oxford) 2007;46(4):608–11.

34. Kapetanovic MC, Saxne T, Sjöholm A, et al. Influence of methotrexate, TNF blockers and prednisolone on antibody responses to pneumococcal polysaccharide vaccine in patients with rheumatoid arthritis. Rheumatology (Oxford) 2006; 45(1):106–11.

35. Kapetanovic MC, Roseman C, Jönsson G, et al. Antibody response is reduced following vaccination with 7-valent conjugate pneumococcal vaccine in adult methotrexate-treated patients with established arthritis, but not those treated with tumor necrosis factor inhibitors. Arthritis Rheum 2011;63(12): 3723–32.

36. Elkayam O, Bashkin A, Mandelboim M, et al. The effect of infliximab and timing of vaccination on the humoral response to influenza vaccination in patients with rheumatoid arthritis and ankylosing spondylitis. Semin Arthritis Rheum 2010; 39(6):442–7.

37. Salemi S, Picchianti-Diamanti A, Germano V, et al. Influenza vaccine administration in rheumatoid arthritis patients under treatment with TNF alpha blockers: safety and immunogenicity. Clin Immunol 2010;134(2):113–20.

38. Gelinck LB, van der Bijl AE, Beyer WE, et al. The effect of anti-tumour necrosis factor alpha treatment on the antibody response to influenza vaccination. Ann Rheum Dis 2008;67(5):713–6.

39. Kaine JL, Kivitz AJ, Birbara C, et al. Immune responses following administration of influenza and pneumococcal vaccines to patients with rheumatoid arthritis receiving adalimumab. J Rheumatol 2007;34(2):272–9.

40. Visvanathan S, Keenan GF, Baker DG, et al. Response to pneumococcal vaccine in patients with early rheumatoid arthritis receiving infliximab plus methotrexate or methotrexate alone. J Rheumatol 2007;34(5):952–7.

41. Elkayam O, Caspi D, Reitblatt T, et al. The effect of tumor necrosis factor blockade on the response to pneumococcal vaccination in patients with rheumatoid arthritis and ankylosing spondylitis. Semin Arthritis Rheum 2004;33(4):283–8.

42. Heijstek MW, Scherpenisse M, Groot N, et al. Immunogenicity and safety of the bivalent HPV vaccine in female patients with juvenile idiopathic arthritis: a prospective controlled observational cohort study. Ann Rheum Dis 2014;73(8):1500–7.

43. Gisbert JP, Villagrasa JR, Rodríguez-Nogueiras A, et al. Efficacy of hepatitis B vaccination and revaccination and factors impacting on response in patients with inflammatory bowel disease. Am J Gastroenterol 2012;107(10):1460–6.

44. Salinas GF, De Rycke L, Barendregt B, et al. Anti-TNF treatment blocks the induction of T cell-dependent humoral responses. Ann Rheum Dis 2013;72(6):1037–43.

45. Zhang J, Delzell E, Xie F, et al. The use, safety, and effectiveness of herpes zoster vaccination in individuals with inflammatory and autoimmune diseases: a longitudinal observational study. Arthritis Res Ther 2011;13(5):R174.

46. Insinga RP, Itzler RF, Pellissier JM, et al. The incidence of herpes zoster in a United States administrative database. J Gen Intern Med 2005;20(8):748–53.

47. Yun H, Xie F, Delzell E, et al. Risks of herpes zoster in patients with rheumatoid arthritis according to biologic disease-modifying therapy. Arthritis Care Res (Hoboken) 2015;67(5):731–6.

48. Oliveira AC, Mota LM, Santos-Neto LL, et al. Seroconversion in patients with rheumatic diseases treated with immunomodulators or immunosuppressants, who were inadvertently revaccinated against yellow fever. Arthritis Rheumatol 2015; 67(2):582–3.

49. Scheinberg M, Guedes-Barbosa LS, Mangueira C, et al. Yellow fever revaccination during infliximab therapy. Arthritis Care Res (Hoboken) 2010;62(6):896–8.

50. Arad U, Tzadok S, Amir S, et al. The cellular immune response to influenza vaccination is preserved in rheumatoid arthritis patients treated with rituximab. Vaccine 2011;29(8):1643–8.

51. Rehnberg M, Brisslert M, Amu S, et al. Vaccination response to protein and carbohydrate antigens in patients with rheumatoid arthritis after rituximab treatment. Arthritis Res Ther 2010;12(3):R111.

52. van Assen S, Holvast A, Benne CA, et al. Humoral responses after influenza vaccination are severely reduced in patients with rheumatoid arthritis treated with rituximab. Arthritis Rheum 2010;62(1):75–81.

53. Oren S, Mandelboim M, Braun-Moscovici Y, et al. Vaccination against influenza in patients with rheumatoid arthritis: the effect of rituximab on the humoral response. Ann Rheum Dis 2008;67(7):937–41.

54. Crnkic Kapetanovic M, Saxne T, Jönsson G, et al. Rituximab and abatacept but not tocilizumab impair antibody response to pneumococcal conjugate vaccine in patients with rheumatoid arthritis. Arthritis Res Ther 2013;15(5):R171.
55. Bingham CO, Looney RJ, Deodhar A, et al. Immunization responses in rheumatoid arthritis patients treated with rituximab: results from a controlled clinical trial. Arthritis Rheum 2010;62(1):64–74.
56. Ribeiro AC, Laurindo IM, Guedes LK, et al. Abatacept and reduced immune response to pandemic 2009 influenza A/H1N1 vaccination in patients with rheumatoid arthritis. Arthritis Care Res (Hoboken) 2013;65(3):476–80.
57. Mori S, Ueki Y, Hirakata N, et al. Impact of tocilizumab therapy on antibody response to influenza vaccine in patients with rheumatoid arthritis. Ann Rheum Dis 2012;71(12):2006–10.
58. Bingham CO, Rizzo W, Kivitz A, et al. Humoral immune response to vaccines in patients with rheumatoid arthritis treated with tocilizumab: results of a randomised controlled trial (VISARA). Ann Rheum Dis 2015;74(5):818–22.
59. Mori S, Ueki Y, Akeda Y, et al. Pneumococcal polysaccharide vaccination in rheumatoid arthritis patients receiving tocilizumab therapy. Ann Rheum Dis 2013; 72(8):1362–6.
60. Chalmers A, Scheifele D, Patterson C, et al. Immunization of patients with rheumatoid arthritis against influenza: a study of vaccine safety and immunogenicity. J Rheumatol 1994;21(7):1203–6.
61. Fischer L, Gerstel PF, Poncet A, et al. Pneumococcal polysaccharide vaccination in adults undergoing immunosuppressive treatment for inflammatory diseases–a longitudinal study. Arthritis Res Ther 2015;17:151.
62. Kernéis S, Launay O, Ancelle T, et al. Safety and immunogenicity of yellow fever 17D vaccine in adults receiving systemic corticosteroid therapy: an observational cohort study. Arthritis Care Res (Hoboken) 2013;65(9):1522–8.
63. Lok AS, McMahon BJ. Chronic hepatitis B: update 2009. Hepatology 2009;50(3): 661–2.
64. Sorrell MF, Belongia EA, Costa J, et al. National Institutes of Health consensus development conference statement: management of hepatitis B. Ann Intern Med 2009;150(2):104–10.
65. Weinbaum CM, Williams I, Mast EE, et al. Recommendations for identification and public health management of persons with chronic hepatitis B virus infection. MMWR Recomm Rep 2008;57(RR-8):1–20.

Barriers to Immunizations and Strategies to Enhance Immunization Rates in Adults with Autoimmune Inflammatory Diseases

CrossMark

Elizabeth Kirchner, MSN[a],*, Victoria Ruffing, RN-BC, CCRP[b]

KEYWORDS

- Immunization • Barriers • Autoimmune inflammatory disease • Adult

KEY POINTS

- Barriers to immunization have existed for as long as immunization.
- Immunization rates in adults are below target.
- Barriers to immunization must be identified and strategies developed to increase immunization rates.
- All health care providers, both primary and specialty, should assess patients for immunization needs.
- Specialty providers, including rheumatologists, should offer vaccines appropriate to immunocompromised patients.

INTRODUCTION AND BRIEF HISTORY OF BARRIERS TO IMMUNIZATION

It seems that for as long as humans have practiced immunization, there have been barriers to it. Evidence suggests that immunizations have been used to prevent disease for almost 1000 years; the variolation technique, used to prevent smallpox, was likely developed in the 1100s and used in Turkey, Africa, China, and parts of Europe.[1] In many of these areas those in favor of variolation were challenged by traditional healers who believed that smallpox was a natural way for the body to expel "bad humors" and religious leaders who believed that attempting to prevent smallpox would anger gods or goddesses.[2] Nevertheless, the practice of variolation spread to

The authors declare no conflicts of interest relevant to the topics of this article.
[a] Department of Rheumatic and Immunologic Disease, Cleveland Clinic, 9500 Euclid Avenue Desk A-50, Cleveland, OH 44195, USA; [b] Johns Hopkins Arthritis Center, Mason F. Lord Center Tower, 5200 Eastern Avenue, Suite 4100, Baltimore, MD 21224, USA
* Corresponding author.
E-mail address: kirchne@ccf.org

Rheum Dis Clin N Am 43 (2017) 15–26
http://dx.doi.org/10.1016/j.rdc.2016.09.004
0889-857X/17/© 2016 Elsevier Inc. All rights reserved.

Western Europe and North America in the 1700s, but there, too, it was not without controversy. Even then, when smallpox outbreaks routinely caused significant illness, disfigurement, and death, there were barriers to immunization of both children and adults. Some physicians saw the benefit of variolation but attempted to corner the market by intentionally making the process more difficult than it needed to be; by cultivating the belief that variolation required deep cuts and significant bloodletting, they ensured that those seeking immunization would have to pay for a major procedure versus the light scratch and inoculation that historically had been performed at times even by amateurs.[3] The major objections to variolation in the Puritan colonies during the early to mid-1700s were on both medical and religious grounds; ministers weighed in on the debate and had significant influence over their congregations. Although many Puritan ministers supported variolation (including, most famously, Cotton Mather [**Fig. 1**]), those who opposed it were often able to prevent their members from seeking immunization. One way to combat this barrier was to instruct non-physicians on how to immunize themselves and their children (thereby overcoming 2 barriers: cost and stigma); Benjamin Franklin encouraged his friend, the English physician William Heberden, to write a pamphlet in 1759 entitled, "Some Account of the Success of Inoculation for the Small-Pox in England and America: Together with Plain Instructions, By which any Person may be enabled to perform the Operation, and conduct the Patient through the Distemper." The pamphlets were distributed for free in the American colonies.[4] By 1775 the benefit to national security seen by preventing smallpox was recognized, and George Washington ordered that all troops in the Continental Army be variolated. This helped spread acceptance of the practice until it was eventually replaced by the safer form of immunization, vaccination.[4]

During the 1721 Boston smallpox epidemic, Puritan minister Cotton Mather urged a local physician to use variolation to prevent the spread of the epidemic. The practice,

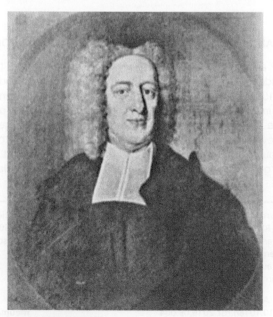

Fig. 1. Cotton Mather, FRS (1663-1728).

although successful, was not without controversy: a grenade was thrown through a window of Mather's house. About the negative reaction, Mather wrote, "I never saw the Devil so let loose upon any occasion. The people who made the loudest Cry...had a very Satanic Fury acting them.... Their common Way was to rail and rave, and wish Death or other Mischiefs, to them that practis'd, or favour'd this devilish Invention."[5]

Since the transition from variolation to vaccination, the science of immunization has grown from the ability to prevent smallpox to the ability now to offer protection against 20 diseases.[6] Despite advances made in vaccinology, however, barriers to immunization have prevented vaccines from being as protective as they could be. This article reviews topics relevant to immunizations in the adult autoimmune inflammatory disease population:

- Recommended immunizations
- The current status of immunization
- Barriers to immunization
- Possible strategies to overcome barriers to immunization

RECOMMENDED IMMUNIZATIONS

The Advisory Council on Immunization Practices (ACIP), a division of the Centers for Disease Control and Prevention (CDC), releases updates to both childhood and adult vaccine schedules annually.[7] Diseases that are represented in the 2016 recommended vaccine schedule for adults are listed in **Box 1**.

Not every patient is a candidate for every vaccine; for example, patients who have been exposed to and developed a natural immunity for hepatitis A or hepatitis B do not require vaccination. Furthermore, not all of these vaccines are appropriate for adults with autoimmune inflammatory disease. The ACIP provides guidelines

---

Box 1
Diseases targeted in the 2016 Advisory Council on Immunization Practices adult vaccine schedule

- Influenza
- Tetanus
- Diphtheria
- Pertussis
- Chickenpox
- Genital warts and genital, anal, and oropharyngeal cancers
- Shingles
- Measles
- Mumps
- Rubella
- Pneumonia
- Hepatitis A
- Hepatitis B
- Meningitis

regarding timing, frequency, sequencing, contraindications, and special populations for each vaccine. Special attention must be given to the footnotes on each schedule, which provide further details and guidance for each vaccine and each special population. Patients with autoimmune inflammatory disease on greater than 20 mg prednisone per day (or the equivalent) or biologics are considered immunocompromised and should follow the schedule for adults with immunocompromising conditions. **Table 1** is an abbreviated version of the 2016 ACIP recommendations for healthy adults and adults with immunocompromising conditions intended only to point out the differences between the 2 groups in the broadest sense; the full schedule with footnotes should always be referenced to ensure that the provider's information is accurate and up to date. In addition, the ACIP frequently makes changes between yearly updates and communicates this to providers and the public via the *Morbidity and Mortality Weekly Report*, press releases, and the CDC Web site.

The recommendations for immunizing patients with autoimmune inflammatory disease can be confusing; both the American College of Rheumatology and the European League Against Rheumatism periodically publish their own recommendations to provide further guidance to rheumatologists and rheumatology practitioners. In addition, articles are frequently published in rheumatology journals addressing the issues surrounding vaccinating patients with autoimmune inflammatory disease (for 2 recent examples, see Westra and colleagues[8] and Friedman and Wintrhop[9]).

Research into new vaccines is ongoing; in 2012 there were approximately 300 vaccine trials conducted, 170 of them for infectious diseases.[10] As research continues into new vaccines as well as the long-term efficacy and safety of current vaccines, rheumatology practitioners can expect that vaccine schedules and recommendations will continue to evolve, which raises the questions, How are we doing with the vaccines we already have? Are we adequately protecting our patients? and If not, what

Table 1
Abbreviated 2016 Advisory Council on Immunization Practices recommendations

Vaccine	Frequency over Adult Years	
	Healthy	Immunocompromised
Influenza	1 dose annually	1 dose annually
Tetanus/diphtheria/pertussis	Substitute Tdap for Td once, then Td booster every 10 years	Substitute Tdap for Td once, then Td booster every 10 y
Varicella	2 doses	Contraindicated
Human papillomavirus	3 doses	3 doses
Zoster	1 dose	Contraindicated
Measles/mumps/rubella	1–2 doses	Contraindicated
Pneumococcal 13-valent conjugate	1 dose	1 dose
Pneumococcal polysaccharide	1–2 doses	1–3 doses
Hepatitis A	2–3 doses	2–3 doses
Hepatitis B	3 doses	3 doses
Meningococcal 4-valent conjugant or polysaccharide	1+ doses	1+ doses
Meningococcal B	2–3 doses	2 or 3
Haemophilus influenzae type B	1 or 3 doses	1–3 doses

Abbreviations: Td, tetanus/diphtheria; Tdap, tetanus/diphtheria/pertussis.

are the barriers to immunization that we can address to improve vaccination rates in patients?

RECENT IMMUNIZATION RATES IN THE UNITED STATES

In 2010 the US Department of Health and Human Services (DHHS) updated the National Vaccine Plan, which was originally drafted in 1994. The 2010 update had 5 goals: develop new and improved vaccines; enhance the vaccine safety system; support informed vaccine decision-making; ensure a stable supply to, access of, and better use of recommended vaccines in the United States; and increase global prevention of death and disease through safe and effective vaccination.[11] Through social media, outreach to primary care providers, continuing medical education programs, and publication of recommended standards of practice, the DHHS has been attempting to increase awareness of and involvement in the promotion of adult immunization. They also focus on assisting public health departments with reimbursement issues to allow them to be able to afford to offer more vaccines to residents. The DHHS 2014 annual report (using 2011–2012 data) showed small but meaningful increases in adult vaccination rates for some specific vaccines and populations (**Fig. 2**) just 2 years into their campaign.

For a more detailed examination of current immunization rates, including a breakdown of special populations, the CDC provides thorough annual reports, which have a wealth of information. Through in-person (National Health Interview Survey), telephone (Behavioral Risk Factor Surveillance System), and Internet (panel surveys) interviews and surveys as well as the Pregnancy Risk Assessment Monitoring System and the Center for Medicare & Medicaid Services Minimum Data Set, the CDC calculates yearly vaccination rates for many adult vaccines. The most recent analysis available is from 2014 and is summarized in **Table 2**.

The CDC Web site provides further analysis of vaccination rates by breaking them down by race/ethnicity, high-risk status, and geographic location. With all these data, along with the multiagency DHHS National Vaccine Plan, it would seem that barriers to immunization might be easily identified and overcome; unfortunately, such is not the case. The rates from the most recent report, although slightly improved over previous years, are still low and well below national goals (**Table 3**).

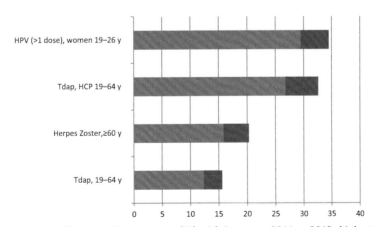

Fig. 2. Selected adult vaccination coverage (%) with increases 2011 to 2012. (*Adapted from* Department of Health & Human Services. The annual report of the state of the national vaccine plan. 2014. Available at: http://www.hhs.gov/nvpo/vacc_plan/annual-report-2014/na tionalvaccineplan2014.pdf.)

Table 2
Centers for Disease Control and Prevention vaccination rates for adults

Vaccination	Population	Rate (%)
Influenza	Age 19 or older	43.2
Pneumococcal (ever)	Age 19–64, high risk	20.3
Pneumococcal (ever)	Age 65 or older	61.3
Tetanus (within 10 y)	Age 19 or older	62.2
Tetanus, including pertussis (within 9 y)	Age 19 or older	20.1
Hepatitis A (2 doses, ever)	Age 19 or older	9.0
Hepatitis B (3 doses, ever)	Age 19 or older	24.5
Shingles (ever)	Age 60 or older	27.9
Human papillomavirus (1 dose, ever)	Females age 19–26	40.2
Human papillomavirus (1 dose, ever)	Males age 19–26	8.2

Adapted from Surveillance of vaccination coverage among adult populations — United States, 2014. Surveillance Summaries 2016;65(1):1–36.

STRATEGIES TO ENHANCE IMMUNIZATIONS IN ADULTS WITH AUTOIMMUNE INFLAMMATORY DISEASES
Basic Challenges

Factors contributing to low vaccination rates include cost and reimbursement to the provider as well as the patient, lack of vaccine requirements for adults (in contrast to the pediatric population, for whom vaccines are required for entry in daycare and school), limited tools for providers to implement a vaccine program, and lack of awareness of adults to recognize the importance of vaccines. The National Vaccine Advisory Committee recommends all health care providers assess patients for vaccination needs. Both primary and specialty care providers should offer appropriate vaccines at each encounter. Should the provider not stock the needed vaccine(s), the patient should be referred to a provider who does.[12] Additionally, all vaccines should be documented.

Interventions — Improving the Rate of Vaccinations

In 1996 the DHHS established the Community Preventive Services Task Force to identify population health interventions that are scientifically proved to save lives, increase lifespans, and improve quality of life. The task force is an independent, nonfederal,

Table 3
Adult vaccination, 2012 coverage and 2020 targets

Vaccine, Target Population	2012 (%)	2020 Target (%)
Influenza, ≥18 y	39	70
Influenza, health care personnel	62	90
Pneumonia, ≥65 y	60	90
Pneumonia, high risk, 19–64 y	20	60
Shingles, ≥60 y	20	30
Hepatitis B vaccine, health care personnel	64	90

From National Vaccine Program Office (2015) National adult immunization plan. Available at: http://www.hhs.gov/nvpo/national_adult_immunization_plan_draft.pdf.

Table 4
Centers for Disease Control and Prevention Recommendations for improving immunizations across the lifespan

Recommendation	Definition	Findings
Patient reminder and recall	Remind members of a target population that vaccinations are due (reminders) or late (recall). Reminders and recalls differ in content and are delivered by various methods—telephone, letter, postcard, text messages, or other.	**Strong evidence** Findings should be broadly applicable to all patient populations, in both clinical and community settings, and for the range of vaccines and delivery methods.
Patient rewards	Client or family incentive rewards are used to motivate people to obtain recommended vaccinations. Rewards may be monetary or nonmonetary. Rewards are typically small (eg, food vouchers, gift cards, lottery prizes, baby products).	**Sufficient evidence** Findings should be broadly applicable to all patient populations, in both clinical and community settings, and for the range of vaccines and delivery methods.

Patient education	Clinic-based client education interventions target individuals or groups served in a medical or public health clinical setting. Educational approaches include the use of brochures, videotapes, posters, vaccine information statements, and face-to-face sessions to inform clients and motivate them to obtain recommended vaccinations in the clinic.	• **Insufficient evidence** of education alone
		• **Strong evidence** when combined with one of the following:
		  ○ Reduced client out-of-pocket costs
		  ○ Home visits
		  ○ Provider reminders
		  ○ Standing orders
		  ○ Provider assessment and feedback

Standing orders	Authorization of nurses, pharmacists, and other health care personnel (where allowed by state law) to assess a client's immunization status and administer vaccinations according to a protocol approved by an institution, physician, or other authorized provider.	**Strong evidence** of effectiveness in increasing vaccination rates among adults and children when used alone or with additional interventions and across a range of settings and populations.
Home visits	Home visitors assess clients' vaccination status, discuss the importance of recommended vaccinations, and either provide vaccinations to clients in their homes or refer them to available immunization services. Home visits may be conducted by vaccination providers (eg, nurses) or others (eg, social workers, community health workers).	**Strong evidence** of effectiveness in increasing vaccination rates among adults and children.
Community-wide education	Community-wide education disseminates information to most or all of a target population in a geographic area with the goal of motivating individuals to seek recommended vaccinations. Materials and messages typically focus on the importance of vaccinations and inform people when and where they can get vaccinated. These interventions may also provide information to vaccination providers in the community.	**Insufficient evidence** to determine the effectiveness of community-wide education when implemented alone in increasing vaccination rates or reducing rates of vaccine preventable illness.

Data from The community guide. Increasing appropriate vaccination: task force recommendations and findings. Available at: http://www.thecommunityguide.org/vaccines/index.html. Accessed May 8, 2016.

unpaid panel of public health and prevention experts that provides evidence-based findings and recommendations about community preventive services, programs, and policies to improve health. Its members represent a broad range of research, practice, and policy expertise in community preventive services, public health, health promotion, and disease prevention.[13] The 15 task force members are appointed by the director of the CDC. Task force members serve 5-year terms, with possible extensions to maintain a full scope of expertise, complete specific work, and ensure consistency of task force recommendations.

The CDC provides administrative, research, and technical support for the Community Preventive Services Task Force. Support is provided by the Community Guide Branch; Division of Public Health Information Dissemination; Center for Surveillance, Epidemiology and Laboratory Services, Office of Public Health Scientific Services; CDC.

Through rigorous systematic literature reviews, the task force has produced recommendations for improving immunizations across the lifespan (**Table 4**).

Social media outlets, such as Facebook and Twitter, offer new and novel ways to potentially improve patient outcomes. There is some evidence that using mobile phone messaging focused on preventative health care may hold some success. This can be used with or without an automated system.[14] Patient portals, systems tied to the electronic health record, generally have good reviews by patients who use them, but patient race, ethnicity, and literacy seem to be barriers to wider use.[15]

In the United States and Canada, pharmacists have taken a more active role in the provision of vaccines. Pharmacists are capable of explaining risks and benefits of vaccines and hold inexpensive seasonal flu vaccine clinics in pharmacies and larger stores where a pharmacy is present, for example, grocery stores. The acceptance and promotion of this alternative to the provider's office may improve immunization rates.[16]

Much research has been conducted in rheumatology clinics regarding how to improve immunization rates in immunosuppressed patients. At the 2014 American College of Rheumatology meeting alone there were more than 10 abstracts related to this subject. Interventions from several of those abstracts are summarized in **Table 5**. Many of them incorporate the use of electronic medical records in both the use of prompts and order sets as interventions. A recent quality improvement

Table 5
Interventions to improve immunization rates in rheumatology clinics

Vaccine Target	Intervention	Change in Vaccination Rate	American College of Rheumatology 2014 Abstract No.
PPSV-23	EMR best practice alert	+7%	1344
PPSV-23, PCV-13	Education, standing orders	PPSV-23 + 6.8% PCV-13 + 30%	1345
PPSV-23, HZVx	Performance reports, best practice alerts, patient outreach	PPSV-23 + 18.5% HZVx + 2.2%	1346
HZVx	Best practice alerts	HZVx + 5.8%	1348
HZVx	Screening tool in prior authorization form	HZVx + 17%	1349

Abbreviations: EMR, electronic medical record; HZVx, herpes zoster vaccine; PCV-13, pneumococcal conjugate vaccine; PPSV-23 pneumococcal polysaccharide vaccine.

study at the Brigham and Women's Hospital (Boston, Massachusetts)[17] demonstrated that vaccine adherence improves when staff and specialists integrate improvement strategies into their workflow. Three interventions were initiated in 4 specialties—allergy, infectious disease, pulmonary, and rheumatology. Nurse-driven model, patient letters, and physician reminders each showed positive results in improving vaccination rates. Data were collected through the electronic medical record. Physicians, nurses, and office staff reinforced patient education surrounding vaccines. Pneumococcal vaccination rates in the rheumatology cohort rose from 50% in 2009 to 87% in 2015.

Box 2
Common patient questions and suggested answers regarding vaccines in rheumatology practice

Question: Will the flu shot make me flare?

Answer: I cannot promise you that it won't make you flare, but that is really rare. If you do flare, we can take care of that for you. (There is a lack of evidence tying immunizations to flare although it has been seen.)

Question: If I get a flu shot, will I get the flu?

Answer: The flu shot does not have any live flu virus in it. If you get a cold or other virus, it is not from the shot. It takes 2 to 3 weeks for the flu shot to work, so if you get the flu, it means you were exposed to the flu either before you got your shot or soon after. The flu shot is made from killed germs. Your body reacts to the germs and makes something called antibodies. The antibodies will kill the flu germs if you ever get exposed to them.

Question: Why should I get the flu shot? I have never gotten the flu before.

Answer: Since your immune system does not work well, you may be more likely to catch something. Getting the flu shot gives you the best chance of avoiding the flu. We want you to have all the protection you can get. Even if you still get the flu after the shot, the vaccine may keep you from getting a flu-related heart attack or making any lung diseases worse.

Question: How do I know the vaccine is safe?

Answer: The United States has a vaccine safety program. All vaccines are tested for safety and checked by the Federal Drug Administration and CDC.

Question: What are the side effects of the vaccine?

Answer: The most common side effects include soreness, redness, or swelling at the site where you got the shot. Severe side effects, like an allergic reaction, are very rare.

Question: Should I get a shingles vaccine?

Answer 1: Yes. Because your immune system does not work well, you are more likely to get shingles than other people. At some point in your future we may treat you with a drug called a biologic, and it is important to get your shingles vaccine *before* we do that.

Answer 2: No. You are on (insert name of biologic); you cannot get the shingles vaccine. The current shingles vaccine is made from the live virus and may cause you to get shingles. Researchers are looking into both a nonlive shingles vaccine and also ways to give the live shingles vaccine to people on biologics. But right now the recommendation is to not get it while you are on a biologic.

Question: Will the flu shot prevent the stomach flu?

Answer: Nausea, vomiting, and diarrhea are not the flu. Those symptoms are caused by many different types of viruses and parasites. The flu is a respiratory illness, not a stomach illness. The flu vaccine will not prevent you from getting a stomach bug.

Table 6 Free clinic resources	
Resource	**Description**
http://www.cdc.gov/flu/pdf/freeresources/ general/cannot-miss-work-flu-flyer.pdf	Colorful flyer can be downloaded.
http://www.cdc.gov/flu/pdf/freeresources/ healthcare/stickers-patient.pdf	These downloadable stickers can be printed on laser and inkjet printers. They fit Avery label numbers: 5160, 5260, 5920, 5960, 5970, 5971, 5972, 5979, 5980, 6460, 8160, 8250, 8460, 8660, 8920, 8930.
http://www.cdc.gov/vaccines/hcp/vis/index. html	Vaccine information statements – required by federal law to be given to the patient prior to every dose of specific vaccines
http://www.niaid.nih.gov/topics/Flu/ Documents/sick.pdf	Poster listing cold vs flu symptoms
http://www.hopkinsarthritis.org/arthritis-news/vaccinations-for-the-arthritis-patient/	Video discussing need for vaccinations in patients with rheumatic diseases

PATIENT FEARS AND CONCERNS

Addressing patient fears and concerns surrounding vaccines cannot be discounted. The Patient Protection and Affordable Care Act of 2010, Title V, defines health literacy as the degree to which an individual has the capacity to obtain, communicate, process, and understand basic health information and services to make appropriate health decisions. A large piece of communicating necessary information to patients is to use plain language. Plain language makes it easier for patients to understand and use health information.

Rheumatologists well understand the need for vaccines in the immunocompromised population. Answering patient concerns in plain language may help patients in making an informed decision (**Box 2**, **Table 6**).

SUMMARY

1. Barriers to immunization have existed for as long as immunization.
2. Immunization rates in adults are below target.
3. Barriers to immunization must be identified and strategies developed to increase immunization rates.
4. All health care providers, both primary and specialty, should assess patients for immunization needs.
5. Specialty providers, including rheumatologists, should offer vaccines appropriate to immunocompromised patients.
6. Recommendations for improving immunization adherence may include electronic reminders and social media.
7. The use of screening, best practice alerts, and standing orders may improve immunization rates in rheumatology practices.
8. Patient education using plain language may improve patient decision making regarding immunizations.

DISCUSSION

The fact that barriers exist, and have existed for centuries, is well-documented in the world of immunization. In addition, in the broadest sense, the types of barriers have not changed over the past many centuries: fear, economics, access, and social pressures. What has changed, especially during the era of biologics, is the knowledge among rheumatologists that patients with autoimmune inflammatory diseases are particularly vulnerable to more frequent and more severe cases of vaccine-preventable illnesses. There is a growing sense of urgency and responsibility to protect patients; however, care must be taken to protect them in the safest manner possible. Issues of timing and education are of paramount importance when it comes to vaccinating patients in the rheumatology clinic. It is the authors' hope that this issue of *Rheumatic Disease Clinics of North America* will empower and inspire rheumatologists and rheumatology practitioners to incorporate immunization and immunization awareness into their daily practice.

REFERENCES

1. Immunization Action Coalition. Available at: http://www.immunize.org/timeline/. Accessed April 15, 2016.
2. Williams G. Angel of death: the story of smallpox. Basingstoke (United Kingdom): Palgrave Macmillan; 2010.
3. Razzell P. The conquest of smallpox: the impact of inoculation on smallpox mortality in eighteenth century britain. Sussex (United Kingdom): Caliban Books; 1977.
4. The historical medical library of the College of Physicians of Philadelphia. The history of vaccines. Available at: http://www.historyofvaccines.org/content/timelines/all. Accessed April 15, 2016.
5. Glynn I, Glynn J. The life and death of smallpox. New York: Cambridge University Press; 2004.
6. U.S. Dept of Health & Human Services. Available at: http://www.vaccines.gov/diseases/. Accessed April 15, 2016.
7. Centers for disease control & prevention. Adult immunization schedule, adults, 2016. Available at: http://www.cdc.gov/vaccines/schedules/hcp/adult.html. Accessed April 15, 2016.
8. Westra J, Rondaan C, van Assen S, et al. Vaccination of patients with autoimmune inflammatory rheumatic diseases. Nat Rev Rheumatol 2015;11(3):135–45.
9. Friedman MA, Winthrop K. Vaccinations for rheumatoid arthritis. Curr Opin Rheumatol 2016;28(3):330–6.
10. Pharmaceutical research and manufacturers of america. 2014 report "medicines in development for vaccines". Available at: http://www.phrma.org/sites/default/files/pdf/vaccines2012.pdf. Accessed April 15, 2016.
11. U.S. Department of Health & Human Services. National vaccine plan. 2010. Available at: http://www.hhs.gov/nvpo/vacc_plan/. Accessed April 15, 2016.
12. Bridges CB, Coyne-Beasley T, ACIP Adult Immunization Work Group, Centers for Disease Control and Prevention. Advisory Committee on Immunization Practices recommended immunization schedule for adults aged 19 years or older - United States, 2014. MMWR Morb Mortal Wkly Rep 2014;63(5):110–2. Available at: http://www.ncbi.nlm.nih.gov/pubmed/24500291. Accessed April 23, 2016.
13. Community Preventive Services Task Force. Increasing appropriate vaccination. Available at: http://www.thecommunityguide.org/vaccines. Accessed April 23, 2016.
14. Vodopivec-Jamsek V, de Jongh T, Gurol-Urganci I, et al. Mobile phone messaging for preventive health care. Cochrane Database Syst Rev 2012;(12):CD007457.
15. Jenssen BP, Mitra N, Shah A, et al. Using digital technology to engage and communicate with patients: a survey of patient attitudes. J Gen Intern Med 2016;31(1):85–92.

16. MacDougall D, Halperin BA, Isenor J, et al. Routine immunization of adults by pharmacists: attitudes and beliefs of the Canadian public and health care providers. Hum Vaccin Immunother 2016;12(3):623–31.
17. Pennant K, Costa J, Fuhlbrigge A, et al. Improving influenza and pneumococcal vaccination rates in ambulatory specialty practices. Open Forum Infect Dis 2015; 2(4):ofv119.

Opportunistic Infections in Biological Therapy, Risk and Prevention

 CrossMark

Paul A. Bryant, MD[a], John W. Baddley, MD, MSPH[b],*

KEYWORDS

- Opportunistic infection • Biologics • Tuberculosis • Zoster • Histoplasmosis
- Pneumocystosis

KEY POINTS

- The risk of opportunistic infections is increased with use of biological therapies.
- The risk of tuberculosis (TB) is increased with anti–tumor necrosis factor (TNF) therapy, and monoclonal antibodies (infliximab, adalimumab) have a higher risk of TB reactivation than etanercept.
- Anti-TNF therapy and tofacitinib are associated with an increased risk of zoster in patients with immune-mediated inflammatory diseases.

INTRODUCTION

Treatment of immune-mediated inflammatory diseases (IMIDs) with biological therapies has resulted in substantial improvement in patient symptoms and has slowed the natural progression of these often-debilitating conditions. Although these therapies have improved the quality of life for many patients, a consequence of biological therapies has been an increased risk of opportunistic infection (OI). In many patients, depending on the underlying disease, there already may be an increased baseline risk of infection independent of disease-modifying therapy.[1,2] A recent meta-analysis of 70 trials including more than 32,000 patients identified an overall increased risk of OIs at 1.7 excess infections per 1000 patients treated with biologics.[3] After the US Food and Drug Administration (FDA) approved infliximab for the treatment of Crohn disease (CD) in 1998, much of the early knowledge on the risk for OIs in the postmarketing period

Disclosures: P.A. Bryant: none; J.W. Baddley: consulting for Merck, Pfizer. Research grant from BMS.
[a] Division of Infectious Diseases, Department of Medicine, University of Alabama at Birmingham, 1900 University Boulevard, 229 THT, Birmingham, AL 35294-0006, USA; [b] Division of Infectious Diseases, Department of Medicine, Birmingham VA Medical Center, University of Alabama at Birmingham and Medical Service, 1900 University Boulevard, 229 THT, Birmingham, AL 35294-0006, USA
* Corresponding author.
E-mail address: jbaddley@uabmc.edu

has come from spontaneous reporting and relied heavily on point-of-care diagnoses. Since that time, newer biological agents with variable mechanisms of action have been approved for a variety of conditions.

Previous reports have shown an increased risk of OIs, serious infections, and hospitalization among users of biologics.[4–7] The French RATIO (Research Axed on Tolerance of Biotherapies) study evaluated nontuberculosis OI risk in patients on anti–tumor necrosis factor (TNF) therapy for any indication and found that infliximab (odds ratio [OR] 17.6) and adalimumab (OR 10.0) carried an increased risk for OIs compared with etanercept.[8] The US Safety Assessment of Biologic Therapy (SABER) study found a higher rate of nonviral OIs among a large cohort of new users of TNF inhibitors (n = 33,324) versus those initiating therapy with nonbiological disease-modifying antirheumatic drugs (DMARDs).[9] In the study's rheumatoid arthritis (RA) cohort new infliximab users experienced a higher rate of nonviral OIs compared with both nonbiological DMARD users (adjusted hazard ratio [aHR] 2.6) and etanercept users (aHR 2.9).

In contrast, a smaller (n = 570) prospective Japanese study evaluating OI incidence in patients with inflammatory bowel disease (IBD) found no increased risk of OIs among patients on infliximab over a 12-month period but did show a risk with other immuno-suppressants and increasing age.[10] A Japanese anti-TNF agent switch study found increased incidence of OIs in the first year of treatment with TNF inhibitors,[11] similar to findings in a retrospective Spanish study showing an increased risk of OIs in the first year of therapy with infliximab.[12] Additional TNF antagonists, such as certolizumab pegol and golimumab, as well as targeted drugs with differing mechanisms of action, such as belimumab, rituximab, tocilizumab, ustekinumab, abatacept, anakinra, and tofacitinib, have also been studied; but data are limited to controlled trials.[13–16]

A major challenge in studying and defining OI risk lies in providing a workable OI case definition. OIs are often difficult to define, and reaching a consensus definition across studies within the area of biological therapy has proven challenging. Although OIs have been more consistently defined within certain diseases, such as human immunodeficiency virus (HIV) infection,[17] this is not the case for biologics. A recent review sought to define OIs in the setting of biologics and provide case definitions for specific candidate pathogens.[18] Although the investigators did reach consensus, they noted that prior attempts to define OIs with the use of biologics have been inconsistent, resulting in wide-ranging OI risk estimates. Herein, the authors review the risk of OIs in biological therapy, with a focus on several major OIs and the most rigorously studied biologics.

TUBERCULOSIS
Incidence and Drug-Specific Risk

Disease due to Mycobacterium tuberculosis remains a major cause of morbidity and mortality, with an estimated 9.6 million cases of incident tuberculosis (TB) worldwide in 2014 according to the most recent World Health Organization's Global Tuberculosis Report.[19] TB has been increasingly reported in patients receiving treatment with biological therapies for a variety of indications since the early 2000s, emphasizing its importance as an opportunistic pathogen. In 2001, Keane and colleagues[20] reported 70 cases of TB in patients on infliximab received through the FDA Adverse Event Reporting System as of May 2001. Cases developed a median of 12 weeks after initiation of therapy, underscoring the need to screen for latent TB infection (LTBI) and disease, especially in areas of high endemicity.

Early studies from North America and Europe found an increased incidence of TB associated with initiation of anti-TNF-α therapy (**Table 1**).[29–32] Surveillance studies

Table 1 Recent studies of tuberculosis and biological therapy				
Reference, Year	Study Type	Location and Period	Person-Years	TB Rate (per 100,000 Person-Years)
Tubach et al,[21] 2009 RATIO	Prospective cohort	France, 2004–2006	57,711	116.7
Dixon et al,[22] 2010 BSRBR	Prospective cohort	Great Britain, 2001–2008	28,447 (on drug)[a]	95
Kim et al,[23] 2011	Retrospective cohort	South Korea, 2002–2009	1784	561
Lee et al,[24] 2013	Retrospective cohort	South Korea, 2002–2011	1717	519
Winthrop et al,[25] 2013	Retrospective cohort	United States, 2000–2008	20,330	49
Abreu et al,[26] 2013	Retrospective cohort	Portugal, 2001–2012	NR	1337 (INF), 792 (ADA), 405 (ETN)
Yoo et al,[27] 2014	Retrospective cohort	South Korea, 2005–2011	231	1300
Baddley et al,[9] 2014 SABER	Retrospective cohort	United States, 1998–2007	22,275	36
Arkema et al,[28] 2015	Prospective cohort	Sweden, 2002–2011	48,228	39.4

Abbreviations: ADA, adalimumab; BSRBR, British Society for Rheumatology Biologics Register; ETN, etanercept; INF, infliximab; NR, not reported.

[a] The investigators used 2 models to report TB cases. *On drug* refers to TB diagnosis being made while patients are actively receiving TNF inhibitor therapy.

from Spain, based on data from the BIOBADASER (Spanish Society of Rheumatology Database on Biologic Products) database established in 2000 for the long-term follow-up of patients with rheumatic diseases on biological therapy, estimated the incidence of TB associated with infliximab to be 1893 cases per 100,000 patients compared with 21 cases per 100,000 inhabitants.[33] Follow-up studies in 2005 and 2007 reported an overall decrease in incidence after the introduction of official screening recommendations by Spanish health authorities. Importantly, the probability of developing active TB was 7 times higher when guidelines were not followed.[34,35]

In the 2009 French RATIO study,[21] 69 validated TB cases were collected based on spontaneous reporting, with the denominator the estimated number of person-years (py) of receipt of anti-TNF therapy in France from 2004 to 2006. The study included patients being treated for RA, spondyloarthropathies, IBD, psoriasis, and Behçet disease. With regard to specific agents used, 36 patients received infliximab, 28 received adalimumab, and 5 were treated with etanercept. Standardized incidence ratios were higher for the monoclonal antibody (mAb) biological class compared with etanercept. A subsequent case-control analysis identified the use of either infliximab or adalimumab versus etanercept as an independent risk factor for TB.

In 2010, Dixon and colleagues[22] addressed the risk of TB between 3 anti-TNF agents (infliximab, adalimumab, etanercept) in patients with RA. Data were from the British Society for Rheumatology Biologics Register (BSRBR), a prospective observational study. A total of 13,739 patients were included, 3232 in the traditional DMARD cohort and 10,712 in the anti-TNF cohort. Forty cases of active TB were reported in the anti-TNF cohort, whereas no cases were reported in the DMARD cohort. Infliximab and adalimumab were associated with a higher rate of TB (136 and 144 events per 100,000 py, respectively) compared with etanercept (39 events per 100,000 py).

A 2011 Korean study reviewing TB in patients with ankylosing spondylitis (AS) found an increased incidence rate of TB in TNF inhibitor (TNFi)-naïve patients versus the general population. Among the patients with AS, no increase in risk was observed between those who were TNFi-naïve and those exposed to biologics.[23] However, a lower risk of TB was observed among users of etanercept compared with the mAb class. In 2013, Lee and colleagues performed a retrospective, longitudinal cohort study from 2002 to 2011 at a large Korean hospital. Among 509 patients treated with TNF antagonists, 9 (1.8%) developed active TB (incidence rate of 519 per 100,000 py).[24] This finding represented a 6.4 times higher incidence of TB than the general population. This study also reported a lower but significant incidence of non-tuberculous mycobacterial (NTM) lung disease (230.7 per 100,000 py).

A US study by Winthrop and colleagues[25] identified more than 8000 anti-TNF users in the United States, most of which had RA, through automated pharmacy records from 2000 to 2008. Estimated anti-TNF–associated TB incidence rates were 49 per 100,000 py compared with 2.8 per 100,000 py in the general population. A retrospective matched case-control study from Portugal reported 25 cases (out of n = 765) of active TB diagnosed in patients on anti-TNF treatment.[26] As noted elsewhere in the literature, patients with TB were more likely to be receiving infliximab (64% of cases) as compared with adalimumab (24%) and etanercept (3 cases), demonstrating an incidence rate of 1337,792 and 405 per 100,000 py, respectively.

A recent retrospective Korean study evaluated the incidence of TB in patients on anti-TNF therapy within a 6-month period.[27] Of 175 cases reviewed in patients with a variety of IMIDs, TB was diagnosed in 3 patients. Although the incidence of TB was estimated to be 18-fold higher than that of the general population, the investigators noted that this might be an overestimation due to underreporting of TB in the general population.

More recently, a large prospective population-based national cohort study from Sweden reported the risk of TB in biological-naïve (n = 37,982) and biological-exposed (n = 10,800) patients with RA from 2002 to 2011.[28] Each patient with RA was matched with up to 5 general population comparators (n = 175,972). When compared with the general population, the biological-naïve patients with RA had a 4-fold increased risk of incident TB. A 2.5-fold higher risk of TB was observed in the biological-exposed patients compared with those who were biological-naïve.[28]

Prevention

Reactivation of LTBI seems to be the predominant reason for the development of disease in low-prevalence countries, with some studies showing an increased risk at the early initiation of therapy. Abreu and colleagues[26] noted that 17 of 25 cases of active TB identified in their Portuguese cohort had been previously diagnosed with LTBI; a large proportion had some combination of negative screening tests, interferon gamma release assay (IGRA), tuberculin skin testing, or chest radiograph,[26] highlighting that the diagnosis of LTBI is not always straightforward. It is important to note that the likelihood of a false-negative screening test may increase in the setting of active treatment with immunosuppressive therapy, before starting biologics. Early reports about the risk of TB and biological therapy have led to the development of guidelines regarding screening and prophylaxis of TB. In some low-prevalence TB countries, screening guidelines have resulted in a reduction in TB incidence.

NONTUBERCULOUS MYCOBACTERIAL DISEASE

Although TB has been established as an important consequence of immunosuppression due to biological therapies, fewer studies have reported on the increased risk of NTM disease in patients on biologics. In the United States, a country with low background rates of TB, the prevalence of NTM disease seems to be increasing.[36–38] Within the SABER cohort study, approximately 11% of the 80 cases of nonviral OIs reported were due to NTM disease.[9] However, the risk between traditional and biological DMARDs was similar. Although a risk differential may exist between TB and NTM disease, the investigators point out the potential for confounding by indication bias, whereby those at risk for NTM infections (eg, severe lung disease) may not be prescribed biological DMARDs.

Data extracted from the large North American health maintenance organization Kaiser Permanente Northern California (KPNC) estimated a higher risk of NTM disease (74 cases per 100,000 py) in those on TNFi compared with the general population and unexposed patients with RA.[25] It has been suggested that NTM disease may be a more important consideration than TB before starting anti-TNF therapy, especially in countries with low TB prevalence. In this KPNC study, a higher proportion of patients with NTM disease died compared with those developing active TB. This finding could be partly due to increased adherence to TB screening guidelines in recent years, a predisposition to pulmonary NTM among patients with RA, or the difficulty in treating pulmonary NTM disease.[39]

Additional investigation is needed in this area, as NTM disease prevalence increases. No screening guidelines exist for patients at risk for infections due to these organisms, and identifying patients at risk is challenging. Providers must remain vigilant for NTM disease development, especially among aging patients with RA with chronic lung disease. No chemoprophylaxis is currently indicated for prevention.

HERPES ZOSTER
Incidence and Drug-Specific Risk

Herpes zoster (HZ), or shingles, due to the reactivation of latent varicella zoster virus (VZV), remains a burdensome disease with potential for long-term disability due to postherpetic neuralgia (PNH).[40] In the United States, there are approximately 1 million new cases diagnosed each year,[41] with those aged 50 years and older being most affected. National incidence of disease has been estimated to be about 3.2 cases per 1000 py overall, with increasing risk in the aging population.[42] Reactivation of latent VZV has been linked to a diminished varicella-specific cell-mediated immunity in the elderly and immunosuppressed.[16] Multiple studies on the incidence of HZ in those on biological therapy have been reported, with a wide range of findings (**Table 2**).

Initial studies have revealed conflicting data on the risk of HZ in patients with various indications for the use of anti-TNF therapy. A US study of more than 20,000 veterans with RA showed a nonsignificant increased risk of zoster with use of infliximab (hazard ratio [HR] 1.32) compared with DMARDs. There was a protective effect observed for adalimumab (HR 0.53) and etanercept (HR 0.62).[43] Of note, the large percentage (more than 90%) of men in this RA cohort makes comparisons with similar studies challenging. A cohort study of patients with RA from Germany using the RABBIT (Rheumatoide Arthritis: Beobachtung der Biologika-Therapie) registry sought to investigate a potential class effect of the anti-TNF drugs as a whole compared with mAbs as a group, etanercept, and DMARDs.[44] Among 5040 patients with RA, 86 episodes of zoster were identified, with crude incidence rate (IRs) per 1000 patient-years of 11.1, 8.9, and 5.6 for those groups, respectively. In a multivariable analysis, there

Table 2
Recent studies of herpes zoster and biological therapy

Reference, Year	Study Type	Location and Period	Person-Years	HZ Rate
McDonald et al,[43] 2009	Retrospective cohort	United States, 1998–2005	~71,000	10.6/1000 py[a]
Strangfeld et al,[44] 2009 RABBIT	Prospective cohort	Germany, 2001–2006	2588 (ETN), 3524 (INF/ADA)	8.9 (ETN), 11.1 (INF/ADA)/1000 py
Garcia-Doval et al,[45] 2010	Prospective cohort	Spain, 2000–2008	15,389[b]	32/100,000 py[b]
Winthrop et al,[46] 2013	Retrospective cohort	United States, 1998–2007	28,392[c]	10.0/1000 py[c]
Galloway et al,[47] 2013 BSRBR	Prospective cohort	United Kingdom, 2001–2009	17,048[d]	1.6/100 py[d]
Winthrop et al,[16] 2014	Retrospective cohort	United States, 2014	290 (low dose), 290 (high dose)[e]	2.1, 5.2/100 py[e]
Yun et al,[48] 2015[f]	Retrospective cohort	United States, 2006–2011	7614 (ABA), 3611 (RTX), 3135 (INF), 2638 (ADA), 2229 (ETN), 839 (TOC), 774 (CTL), 683 (GOL) (per 100 py)	1.87 (ABA), 2.27 (RTX), 1.02 (INF), 1.74 (ADA), 2.15 (ETN), 2.15 (TOC), 2.45 (CTL), 1.61 (GOL) (per 100 py)

Abbreviations: ABA, abatacept; ADA, adalimumab; CTL, certolizumab; ETN, etanercept; GOL, golimumab; INF, infliximab; RTX, rituximab; TOC, tocilizumab; TOF, tofacitinib.
[a] Rates reported from RA cohort group 3, which included patients on infliximab, adalimumab, and etanercept.
[b] All patients with rheumatic disease exposed to TNF antagonists.
[c] Includes new users of etanercept, infliximab, and adalimumab across all indications.
[d] Includes users of etanercept, infliximab, and adalimumab with RA.
[e] Pooled phase III tofacitinib studies in first 3 months of treatment.
[f] Study compares risk between individual biologics.

was a significantly higher risk of HZ with use of mAb therapy (HR 1.82) compared with DMARDs. No significant association was noted for etanercept (HR 1.32) or the anti-TNF class as a whole (HR 1.63).

Similarly, in a study by Smitten and colleagues,[49] data from US and UK databases revealed a 2-fold increase in HZ risk in a large cohort of patients with RA versus non-RA patients, consistent with prior and more recent studies. A nested case-control analysis showed a slight increase in zoster risk in patients on biological DMARDs (OR 1.54) or conventional DMARDs (OR 1.37) versus no DMARD therapy.

A secondary data analysis was published in 2010 from the Spanish BIOBADASER 2.0 registry and a national hospital discharge database with the aim of estimating the incidence of hospitalization due to VZV infection.[45] Of 106 patients with zoster reported, 5 required hospitalization; all hospitalized patients had exposure to anti-TNF agents. The estimated IR of hospitalizations in the exposed patients was 32 cases per 100,000 patient-years. An analysis of patients with RA showed a higher IR for hospitalization compared with all exposed groups. Although there seemed to be a 10-fold increase in the rate of hospitalization compared with the general population, the absolute rate was small (3 cases per 10,000 py), leading the authors to conclude that the risks of routine immunization with the attenuated zoster vaccine probably outweighed the benefits.

Within the French RATIO registry, a 2012 case-control study was conducted with 24 validated HZ cases in patients on anti-TNF therapy compared with controls on therapy.[50] Although the aim of the study was not to report on HZ incidence given the limited sample size, a multivariable analysis suggested that risk decreased as time from exposure to the drug increased. When comparing HZ risk between infliximab, adalimumab, and etanercept individually, there was no statistically significant increase in risk. However, when comparing the risk between the mAb class as a whole (OR 3.49, $P = .03$) with etanercept, the difference was significant.

A large retrospective cohort and nested case-control study in the United States was conducted that included 108,604 patients (1997–2009) with IBD, either CD, ulcerative colitis, or unspecified IBD.[51] Patients with IBD contributed 364,533 py of observation time. A total of 2677 cases of HZ were identified in the IBD group, with 4340 cases of HZ in the non-IBD population. This finding resulted in an overall incidence rate of 734 cases per 100,000 py versus 437 cases per 100,000 py in the non-IBD cohort (incidence rate ratios [IRR] 1.68). The highest incidence of HZ was in patients with CD older than 60 years of age. In the nested case-control study, comparing patients with IBD diagnosed with and without HZ, a significant number of comorbidities were noted in the HZ group. Adjusted analyses revealed an increased risk of HZ in the IBD population overall treated with anti-TNF agents (OR 1.81), although no comparison was made between drugs of this class. A subanalysis revealed that the highest risk of HZ was with combination therapy with an anti-TNF drug plus thiopurine (OR 3.29).

Another US study in 2013, as part of the SABER initiative, evaluated new users of anti-TNF therapy across multiple cohorts of patients with RA, IBD, and psoriasis-psoriatic arthritis (PsA)-AS, combining data from several institutions.[46] National Medicare/Medicaid enrollees were included, probably accounting for older patients making up a larger percentage of the cohorts overall (20% aged >65 years). A total of 310 HZ cases were identified out of 32,208 new anti-TNF users. Crude incidence rates were 12.1, 11.3, and 4.4 per 1000 py for the RA, IBD, and psoriasis-PsA-AS cohorts, respectively. With 160 cases of HZ identified in the nonbiological DMARD group, the crude IRs were similar, suggesting no increased risk of HZ when comparing treatment initiation with biologics versus DMARDs. Furthermore, analysis of the RA cohort found no significant difference in HZ risk with regard to specific TNFi used, after adjustment for steroid use at baseline and propensity score quintile.

A retrospective, population-based cohort study identified 813 patients in Minnesota diagnosed with RA from 1980 to 1997.[52] The rate of development of HZ in the patients with RA was 12.1 per 1000 py versus 5.4 per 1000 py in the non-RA comparator group. Interestingly, HZ occurred more frequently in those diagnosed in the second half of the study (HR 1.9). A similar finding was noted in the non-RA group, reflecting an increase in HZ diagnoses more recently in the general population. The reason for this is unclear but has been the subject of other investigations.[53,54] In addition, this study found no significant increase in risk of HZ in patients treated with DMARDs or biological therapies but did find risk with corticosteroid use.

In the UK, Galloway and colleagues,[47] using data from the BSRBR, estimated incidence rates of zoster and serious skin and soft tissue infections.[47] Patients with RA on anti-TNF therapy (n = 11,881) and DMARDs (n = 3673) were compared using a follow-up questionnaire performed by both patients and providers up to a 3-year follow-up period. Crude IR of shingles for the anti-TNF cohort was 1.6 per 100 (events per patient-years of follow-up) and 0.8 per 100 for the DMARD cohort. Event rates were higher early on in the treatment courses of both cohorts. With regard to drug-specific risk, infliximab showed the highest risk of zoster compared with adalimumab, whereas etanercept showed no increased risk compared with both mAb therapies combined.

Newer therapies have also been evaluated for HZ risk. In a 2014 study, the nonbiological Janus kinase inhibitor tofacitinib was reported to have a crude IR of 4.4 per 100 py for low-dose treatment, with no difference in incidence in the higher-dose patients with regard to zoster risk.[16] Higher rates were particularly noted in Asia. A more recent study with patients with RA on tofacitinib found an incidence of HZ nearly double that of biologics, including anti-TNF drugs, abatacept, rituximab, and tocilizumab, consistent with prior clinical trial data.[55]

In 2015, a retrospective cohort study using Medicare data from 2006 to 2011 identified patients with RA initiating new treatment with abatacept, adalimumab, certolizumab, etanercept, golimumab, infliximab, rituximab, and tocilizumab. Out of 29,129 new treatment episodes, 423 HZ diagnoses were made. Although the highest rates were reported with certolizumab and lowest for golimumab, the difference among all biologics was not significant, suggesting that HZ risk across biological agents with differing mechanisms of action was similar.[48]

Prevention

In 2005, the Shingles Prevention Study demonstrated a reduction in HZ disease burden by 61.1%, decreased incidence of HZ cases by 51.3%, and a decrease in frequency of post-herpetic neuralgia by 66.5% in those who received the live attenuated Oka/Merck strain VZV vaccine compared with placebo.[56] Use of the live attenuated zoster vaccine (Zostavax) in those on recombinant human immune modulators, namely anti-TNF agents, is contraindicated, although the safety of concurrent use is unknown. This contraindication is based on 2008 recommendations from the Advisory Committee on Immunization Practices (ACIP).[57] Administering the vaccine 4 weeks or more before the initiation or after the discontinuation of TNFi is generally recommended.

A recent study sought to evaluate the risk of HZ in younger patients with certain autoimmune or inflammatory (AI) conditions (7 cohorts total) compared with 2 cohorts: older, healthy controls and those with diabetes.[58] Adjusted incidence rates were highest for the systemic lupus erythematosus cohort (19.9 per 1000 py), followed by IBD and RA. This finding is compared with the IR of 5.3 per 1000 py for the non-AI, nondiabetic older cohort. Although the ACIP currently recommends the zoster vaccine for individuals aged 60 years and older, these findings suggest that younger individuals with certain autoimmune conditions may benefit from vaccination. Clinical trials are currently underway to determine the safety and efficacy of vaccination in these populations.

PNEUMOCYSTOSIS
Incidence and Drug-Specific Risk

The fungus Pneumocystis jiroveci has been increasingly recognized as a cause of opportunistic infections in the immunocompromised host since the 1940s and more recently as an initial indicator of the AIDS epidemic.[59] Although an association between development of Pneumocystis jiroveci pneumonia (PJP) and underlying rheumatic disease has been previously described, increased incidence of PJP with modern biological therapy has also been observed.[60–62] True incidence rates are difficult to determine given the relative rarity of PJP in non-HIV infected patients as well the variability in presentation and methods and sensitivity of diagnostic testing.

Cases of PJP were recognized following the approval of infliximab for IBD in 1998.[63,64] A total of 84 cases had been reported to the FDA's Adverse Event Reporting System as of December 2003, and an analysis of these cases revealed high mortality of 27% (23 deaths). Most patients had RA and were diagnosed with PJP early after treatment initiation with infliximab.[64] Several population-based studies have sought to estimate the incidence of PJP in those treated with TNF inhibitors. In the French RATIO study,[8] 5 cases of PJP were reported from 57,711 patient-years of anti-TNF treatment from 2004 to 2006. In the United States, the SABER study reported retrospectively on OI cases occurring from 1998 to 2007.[9] Case identification relied on claims data from 4 health-insurance entities and was composed of patients on anti-TNF therapy for a variety of indications, such as RA, IBD, psoriasis, psoriatic arthritis, and AS. With 28,493 py of exposure to TNFi, 16 cases of PJP were documented.

Previously, a study by the National Institutes of Health sought to determine any difference over time between rates of PJP in patients with RA from 1996 to 2007.[65] Data were used from the Nationwide Inpatient Sample (consisting of 8 million inpatient hospitalizations and 20% of community hospitals in the United States) and the California Office of Statewide Health Planning and Development, and no significant changes in RA and PJP diagnoses were observed over the study period. However, this may have underestimated incidence as it relied on diagnostic codes submitted to insurers to identify cases of PJP. Similarly, the aforementioned RATIO study possibly underestimated PJP incidence because of the failure to diagnose rather than miscoding. In contrast to the aforementioned studies, Dixon and colleagues[66] found no cases of PJP in the 2006 British registry study. Similarly, a study using data from the CORRONA (The Consortium of Rheumatology Researchers of North America) registry in the United States found a very low incidence of PJP with 0.14 cases per 1000 py.[67]

In Japan, several observational studies reported a higher incidence of PJP in patients on anti-TNF drugs compared with similar studies. Takeuchi and colleagues[68] evaluated patients during the first 6 months of treatment with infliximab and estimated an incidence of 8.8 cases per 1000 patient-years. It is important to note that the diagnosis of PJP was made based on physician assessment and a positive polymerase chain reaction (PCR) for *P jiroveci* DNA from bronchoalveolar lavage sampling in nearly all (21 out of 22) of the reported cases. A study by Koike and colleagues[69] enrolled predominantly patients with RA and analyzed the initial 6 months of therapy with etanercept and estimated an incidence of 4.6 cases per 1000 py, whereas Komano and colleagues[70] found an incidence of 5 cases per 1000 py. These 3 Japanese studies had fewer py contributed to the follow-up period than other published reports[8,9,66,67,71] and also relied more often on diagnosis by PCR, which can be positive in asymptomatic individuals on immunosuppressive therapy. Variability in Japanese testing modalities and a more sensitive case definition may account for the increased incidence, but more studies are needed to reach any further conclusions.

Prevention

There are currently no specific recommendations regarding prophylaxis against PJP in patients being treated with anti-TNF medications. Although studies from the United States and Europe have estimated a low incidence of PJP in this patient population, the observational studies discussed from Japan suggest a higher risk of disease in patients with rheumatic diseases undergoing therapy with TNFi, especially during the early treatment period. Given the discrepancy among these population-based studies, administration of trimethoprim-sulfamethoxazole, the drug of choice for both treatment and prophylaxis in most populations,[17,72] does not seem to be warranted with biologics. Further analysis to identify a subset of patients that may benefit from prophylaxis is challenging given the already low incidence of disease reported.

HISTOPLASMOSIS

Fungal infection due to *Histoplasma capsulatum* has been the most common OI with relation to use of biological therapy. Most cases have been reported among patients receiving TNFi, with infliximab accounting for most cases.[73] Early surveillance reports of histoplasmosis were nearly all from endemic areas and occurred within 1 week to 6 months of the first dose of the biological drug. This finding highlights the importance of increased awareness at treatment initiation, especially in the Midwest, Ohio River Valley, and Southeastern United States.[74–76] One retrospective report found 26 cases of histoplasmosis in patients with RA, with nearly 60% of those patients having been exposed to biologics.[77] Median time from exposure to disease was 15 months, suggesting new exposure.

In a series of 19 patients on TNFi diagnosed with histoplasmosis from 2000 to 2009, most presented with progressive, disseminated disease and most patients (13) were receiving infliximab. Immune reconstitution inflammatory syndrome (IRIS) was considered a potential cause of deterioration in 42% of patients in whom histoplasmosis was diagnosed, antifungal therapy was started, and TNFi drugs were discontinued. All 19 patients in the series recovered. The investigators noted that although the FDA suggests discontinuing anti-TNF therapy after histoplasmosis is diagnosed, it is unknown whether or not this increases IRIS risk.[78]

A more recent review of 98 cases of histoplasmosis complicating TNFi therapy generally found favorable disease outcomes during a median follow-up period of 32 months (1–120 months).[79] Mortality was reported at 3.2%, which is lower compared with rates reported in solid organ transplant recipients. The investigators concluded that it was reasonable to consider resuming TNFi treatment in most individuals who have been treated for histoplasmosis without evidence of residual disease or detectable histoplasma antigen.

True incidence of histoplasmosis is difficult to estimate given the regional variability of disease and relatively low number of reported cases. Within the US SABER study, only 9 cases were reported out of more than 33,000 anti-TNF users.[9] No formal guidelines exist for the management of histoplasmosis for those on anti-TNF drugs, but discontinuation of the biologic and prompt initiation of antifungal treatment is generally warranted. Screening or chemoprophylaxis is not currently indicated.

Data on incidence of other endemic mycoses are even more limited. Coccidioidomycosis risk has previously been reported to be higher in infliximab users compared with etanercept in a small series of cases reported on in 2004 from endemic areas.[80] A more recent retrospective chart review recommended that restarting biological therapy after coccidioidomycosis treatment may be safe in some select patients.[81]

SUMMARY

Biological therapy for the treatment of inflammatory conditions has provided great benefit to patients with often-debilitating symptoms. Since the early 2000s, the incidence of opportunistic infections, such as TB, zoster, and PJP, has increased as more biological therapy has been prescribed, although some increase is partly related to heightened awareness. As increasing numbers of biological therapies with distinct mechanisms of action beyond TNF blockade are approved for use, identification of OIs will remain challenging. Population-based studies, national registries, provider vigilance, and screening guidelines will be crucial in establishing and mitigating the risk of OIs going forward.

REFERENCES

1. Wagner UG, Koetz K, Weyand CM, et al. Perturbation of the T cell repertoire in rheumatoid arthritis. Proc Natl Acad Sci U S A 1998;95(24):14447–52.
2. Vallejo AN, Weyand CM, Goronzy JJ. T-cell senescence: a culprit of immune abnormalities in chronic inflammation and persistent infection. Trends Mol Med 2004;10(3):119–24.
3. Kourbeti IS, Ziakas PD, Mylonakis E. Biologic therapies in rheumatoid arthritis and the risk of opportunistic infections: a meta-analysis. Clin Infect Dis 2014; 58:1649–57.
4. Singh JA, Wells GA, Christensen R, et al. Adverse effects of biologics: a network meta-analysis and Cochrane overview. Cochrane Database Syst Rev 2011;(2):CD008794.
5. Marehbian J, Arrighi HM, Hass S, et al. Adverse events associated with common therapy regimens for moderate-to-severe Crohn's disease. Am J Gastroenterol 2009;104(10):2524–33.
6. Toruner M, Loftus EV Jr, Harmsen WS, et al. Risk factors for opportunistic infections in patients with inflammatory bowel disease. Gastroenterology 2008; 134(4):929–36.
7. Smitten AL, Choi HK, Hochberg MC, et al. The risk of hospitalized infection in patients with rheumatoid arthritis. J Rheumatol 2008;35(3):387–93.
8. Salmon-Ceron D, Tubach F, Lortholary O, et al. Drug-specific risk of non-tuberculosis opportunistic infections in patients receiving anti-TNF therapy reported to the 3-year prospective French RATIO registry. Ann Rheum Dis 2011; 70:616–23.
9. Baddley JW, Winthrop KL, Chen L, et al. Non-viral opportunistic infections in new users of tumour necrosis factor inhibitor therapy: results of the Safety Assessment of Biologic ThERapy (SABER) Study. Ann Rheum Dis 2014;73:1942–8.
10. Naganuma M, Kunisaki R, Yoshimura N, et al. A prospective analysis of the incidence of and risk factors for opportunistic infections in patients with inflammatory bowel disease. J Gastroenterol 2013;48:595–600.
11. Nguyen-Khoa BA, Goehring EL Jr, Alexander KA, et al. Risk of significant infection in rheumatoid arthritis patients switching anti-tumor necrosis factor-alpha drugs. Semin Arthritis Rheum 2012;42:119–26.
12. Garcia-Vidal C, Rodriguez-Fernandez S, Teijon S, et al. Risk factors for opportunistic infections in infliximab-treated patients: the importance of screening in prevention. Eur J Clin Microbiol Infect Dis 2009;28:331–7.
13. Salliot C, Dougados M, Gossec L. Risk of serious infections during rituximab, abatacept, and anakinra treatments for rheumatoid arthritis: meta-analyses of randomised placebo-controlled trials. Ann Rheum Dis 2009;68:25–32.
14. Bykerk VP, Cush J, Winthrop K, et al. Update on the safety profile of certolizumab pegol in rheumatoid arthritis: in integrated analysis from clinical trials. Ann Rheum Dis 2015;74:96–103.
15. Winthrop KL, Park S-H, Gul A, et al. Tuberculosis and other opportunistic infections in tofacitinib-treated patients with rheumatoid arthritis. Ann Rheum Dis 2015;0:1–6.
16. Winthrop KL, Yamanaka H, Valdez H, et al. Herpes zoster and tofacitinib therapy in patients with rheumatoid arthritis. Arthritis Rheumatol 2014;66:2675–84.
17. Panel on Opportunistic Infections in HIV-Infected Adults and Adolescents. Guidelines for the prevention and treatment of opportunistic infections in HIV-infected adults and adolescents: recommendations from the Centers for Disease Control and Prevention, the National Institutes of Health, and the HIV

Medicine Association of the Infectious Disease Society of America. Available at: http://aidsinfo.nih.gov/contentfiles/lvguidelines/adult_oi.pdf. Accessed April 10, 2016.

18. Winthrop KL, Novosad SA, Baddley JW, et al. Opportunistic infections and biologic therapies in immune-mediated inflammatory diseases: consensus recommendations for infection reporting during clinical trials and postmarketing surveillance. Ann Rheum Dis 2015;74(12):2107–16.

19. World Health Organization (WHO) Global Tuberculosis Report 2015. Available at: www.who.int/tb/publications/global_report/en. Accessed April 10, 2016.

20. Keane J, Gershon S, Wise RP, et al. Tuberculosis associated with infliximab, a tumor necrosis factor alpha-neutralizing agent. N Engl J Med 2001;345:1098–104.

21. Tubach F, Salmon D, Ravaud P, et al. Risk of tuberculosis is higher with anti-tumor necrosis factor monoclonal antibody therapy than with soluble tumor necrosis factor receptor therapy: the three-year prospective French Research Axed on Tolerance of Biotherapies registry. Arthritis Rheum 2009;60:1884–94.

22. Dixon WG, Hyrich KL, Watson KD, et al. Drug-specific risk of tuberculosis in patients with rheumatoid arthritis treated with anti-TNF therapy: results from the British Society for Rheumatology Biologics Register (BSRBR). Ann Rheum Dis 2010;69:522–8.

23. Kim EM, Uhm WS, Bae SC, et al. Incidence of tuberculosis among Korean patients with ankylosing spondylitis who are taking tumor necrosis factor blockers. J Rheumatol 2011;38:2218–23.

24. Lee SK, Kim SY, Kim EY, et al. Mycobacterial infections in patients treated with tumor necrosis factor antagonists in South Korea. Lung 2013;191:565–71.

25. Winthrop KL, Baxter R, Liu L, et al. Mycobacterial diseases and antitumour necrosis factor therapy in USA. Ann Rheum Dis 2013;72:37–42.

26. Abreu C, Magro F, Santos-Antunes J, et al. Tuberculosis in anti-TNF-alpha treated patients remains a problem in countries with an intermediate incidence: an analysis of 25 patients matched with a control population. J Crohns Colitis 2013;7: e486–92.

27. Yoo IK, Choung RS, Hyun JJ, et al. Incidences of serious infections and tuberculosis among patients receiving anti-tumor necrosis factor-alpha therapy. Yonsei Med J 2014;55:442–8.

28. Arkema EV, Jonsson J, Baecklund E, et al. Are patients with rheumatoid arthritis still at an increased risk of tuberculosis and what is the role of biological treatments? Ann Rheum Dis 2015;74:1212–7.

29. Wolfe F, Michaud K, Anderson J, et al. Tuberculosis infection in patients with rheumatoid arthritis and the effect of infliximab therapy. Arthritis Rheum 2004;50: 372–9.

30. Askling J, Fored CM, Brandt L, et al. Risk and case characteristics of tuberculosis in rheumatoid arthritis associated with tumor necrosis factor antagonists in Sweden. Arthritis Rheum 2005;52:1986–92.

31. Sichletidis L, Settas L, Spyratos D, et al. Tuberculosis in patients receiving anti-TNF agents despite chemoprophylaxis. Int J Tuberc Lung Dis 2006;10:1127–32.

32. Brassard P, Kezouh A, Suissa S. Antirheumatic drugs and the risk of tuberculosis. Clin Infect Dis 2006;43:717–22.

33. Gomez-Reino JJ, Carmona L, Valverde VR, et al. Treatment of rheumatoid arthritis with tumor necrosis factor inhibitors may predispose to significant increase in tuberculosis risk: a multicenter active-surveillance report. Arthritis Rheum 2003; 48:2122–7.

34. Carmona L, Gomez-Reino JJ, Rodriguez-Valverde V, et al. Effectiveness of recommendations to prevent reactivation of latent tuberculosis infection in patients treated with tumor necrosis factor antagonists. Arthritis Rheum 2005;52:1766–72.

35. Gomez-Reino JJ, Carmona L, Angel Descalzo M, et al. Risk of tuberculosis in patients treated with tumor necrosis factor antagonists due to incomplete prevention of reactivation of latent infection. Arthritis Rheum 2007;57:756–61.

36. Cassidy PM, Hedberg K, Saulson A, et al. Nontuberculous mycobacterial disease prevalence and risk factors: a changing epidemiology. Clin Infect Dis 2009;49:e124–9.

37. Winthrop KL, McNelley E, Kendall B, et al. Pulmonary nontuberculous mycobacterial disease prevalence and clinical features; an emerging public health disease. Am J Respir Crit Care Med 2010;182:977–82.

38. Marras TK, Mehta M, Chedore P, et al. Nontuberculous mycobacterial lung infections in Ontario, Canada: clinical and microbiological characteristics. Lung 2010;188:289–99.

39. Griffith DE, Aksamit T, Brown-Elliott BA, et al. An official ATS/IDSA statement: diagnosis, treatment, and prevention of nontuberculous mycobacterial diseases. Am J Respir Crit Care Med 2007;175:367–416.

40. Johnson RW, Rice AS. Clinical practice. Postherpetic neuralgia. N Engl J Med 2014;371:1526–33.

41. Centers for Disease Control and Prevention. Shingles (Herpes Zoster). Available at: http://www.cdc.gov/shingles/about/overview.html. Accessed April 10, 2016.

42. Insinga RP, Itzler RF, Pellissier JM, et al. The incidence of herpes zoster in a United States administrative database. J Gen Intern Med 2005;20:748–53.

43. McDonald JR, Zeringue AL, Caplan L, et al. Herpes zoster risk factors in a national cohort of veterans with rheumatoid arthritis. Clin Infect Dis 2009;48:1364–71.

44. Strangfeld A, Listing J, Herzer P, et al. Risk of herpes zoster in patients with rheumatoid arthritis treated with anti-TNF-alpha agents. JAMA 2009;301:737–44.

45. Garcia-Doval I, Perez-Zafrilla B, Descalzo MA, et al. Incidence and risk of hospitalisation due to shingles and chickenpox in patients with rheumatic diseases treated with TNF antagonists. Ann Rheum Dis 2010;69:1751–5.

46. Winthrop KL, Baddley JW, Chen L, et al. Association between the initiation of anti-tumor necrosis factor therapy and the risk of herpes zoster. JAMA 2013;309:887–95.

47. Galloway JB, Mercer LK, Moseley A, et al. Risk of skin and soft tissue infections (including shingles) in patients exposed to anti-tumour necrosis factor therapy: results from the British Society for Rheumatology Biologics Register. Ann Rheum Dis 2013;72:229–34.

48. Yun H, Xie F, Delzell E, et al. Risks of herpes zoster in patients with rheumatoid arthritis according to biologic disease-modifying therapy. Arthritis Care Res (Hoboken) 2015;67:731–6.

49. Smitten AL, Choi HK, Hochberg MC, et al. The risk of herpes zoster in patients with rheumatoid arthritis in the United States and the United Kingdom. Arthritis Rheum 2007;57:1431–8.

50. Serac G, Tubach F, Marriette X, et al. Risk of herpes zoster in patients receiving anti-TNF-alpha in the prospective French RATIO registry. J Invest Dermatol 2012;132(3 Pt 1):726–9.

51. Long MD, Martin C, Sandler RS, et al. Increased risk of herpes zoster among 108,604 patients with inflammatory bowel disease. Aliment Pharmacol Ther 2013;37:420–9.

52. Veetil BM, Myasoedova E, Matteson EL, et al. Incidence and time trends of Herpes zoster in rheumatoid arthritis: a population-based cohort study. Arthritis Care Res (Hoboken) 2013;65:854–61.

53. Rimland D, Moanna A. Increasing incidence of herpes zoster among veterans. Clin Infect Dis 2010;50:1000–5.

54. Yawn BP, Saddier P, Wollan PC, et al. A population-based study of the incidence and complication rates of herpes zoster before zoster vaccine introduction. Mayo Clin Proc 2007;82:1341–9.

55. Curtis JR, Xie F, Yun H, et al. Real-world comparative risks of herpes virus infections in tofacitinib and biologic-treated patients with rheumatoid arthritis. Ann Rheum Dis 2016;75(10):1843–7.

56. Oxman MN, Lovin MJ, Johnson GR, et al. A vaccine to prevent herpes zoster and postherpetic neuralgia in older adults. N Engl J Med 2005;352:2271–84.

57. Harpaz R, Ortega-Sanchez IR, Seward JF. Prevention of herpes zoster: recommendations of the Advisory Committee on Immunization Practices (ACIP). MMWR Recomm Rep 2008;57(RR-5):1–30.

58. Yun H, Yang S, Chen L, et al. Risk of herpes zoster in auto-immune and inflammatory diseases: implications for vaccination. Arthritis Rheumatol 2016;68(0): 2020–37.

59. Masur H, Michelis MA, Greene JB, et al. An outbreak of community-acquired Pneumocystis carinii pneumonia: initial manifestation of cellular immune dysfunction. N Engl J Med 1981;305:1431–8.

60. Wollner A, Mohle-Boetani J, Lambert RE, et al. Pneumocystis carinii pneumonia complicating low dose methotrexate treatment for rheumatoid arthritis. Thorax 1991;46:205–7.

61. Ward MM, Donald F. Pneumocystis carinii pneumonia in patients with connective tissue diseases: the role of hospital experience in diagnosis and mortality. Arthritis Rheum 1999;42:780–9.

62. Ognibene FP, Shelhamer JH, Hoffman GS, et al. Pneumocystis carinii pneumonia: a major complication of immunosuppressive therapy in patients with Wegener's granulomatosis. Am J Respir Crit Care Med 1995;151(3 Pt 1):795–9.

63. Tai TL, O'Rourke KP, McWeeney M, et al. Pneumocystis carinii pneumonia following a second infusion of infliximab. Rheumatology 2002;41:951–2.

64. Kaur N, Mahl T. Pneumocystis jiroveci (carinii) pneumonia after infliximab therapy: a review of 84 cases. Dig Dis Sci 2007;52:1481–4.

65. Louie G, Wang Z, Ward MW. Trends in hospitalizations for Pneumocystis jiroveci pneumonia among patients with rheumatoid arthritis in the US: 1996–2007. Arthritis Rheum 2010;62:3826–9.

66. Dixon WG, Watson K, Lunt M, et al. Rates of serious infection, including site-specific and bacterial intracellular infection, in rheumatoid arthritis patients receiving anti-tumor necrosis factor therapy: results from the British Society for Rheumatology Biologics Register. Arthritis Rheum 2006;54:2368–76.

67. Greenberg JD, Reed G, Kremer JM, et al. Association of methotrexate and tumour necrosis factor antagonists with risk of infectious outcomes including opportunistic infections in the CORRONA registry. Ann Rheum Dis 2010;69: 380–6.

68. Takeuchi T, Tatsuki Y, Nogami Y, et al. Postmarketing surveillance of the safety profile of infliximab in 5000 Japanese patients with rheumatoid arthritis. Ann Rheum Dis 2008;67:189–94.

69. Koike T, Harigai M, Inokuma S, et al. Postmarketing surveillance of the safety and effectiveness of etanercept in Japan. J Rheumatol 2009;36:898–906.

70. Komano Y, Tanaka M, Nanki T, et al. Incidence and risk factors for serious infection in patients with rheumatoid arthritis treated with tumor necrosis factor inhibitors: a report from the Registry of Japanese Rheumatoid Arthritis Patients for Long term Safety. J Rheumatol 2011;38:1258–64.
71. Lichtenstein GR, Feagan BG, Cohen RD, et al. Serious infection and mortality in patients with Crohn's disease: more than 5 years of follow-up in the TREAT registry. Am J Gastroenterol 2012;107:1409–22.
72. Martin SI, Fishman JA, AST Infectious Diseases Community of Practice. Pneumocystis pneumonia in solid organ transplantation. Am J Transplant 2013;13:272–9.
73. Tsiodoras S, Samonis G, Boumpas DT, et al. Fungal infections complicating tumor necrosis factor alpha blockade therapy. Mayo Clin Proc 2008;83:181–94.
74. Lee J-H, Slifman NR, Gershon SK, et al. Life-threatening histoplasmosis complicating immunotherapy with tumor necrosis factor α antagonists infliximab and etanercept. Arthritis Rheum 2002;46:2565–70.
75. Baddley JW, Winthrop KL, Patkar NM, et al. Geographic distribution of endemic fungal infections among older persons, United States. Emerg Infect Dis 2011;17: 1664–9.
76. U.S. Food and Drug Administration 2008. Manufacturers of TNF-blocker drugs must highlight risk of fungal infections. Available at: http://www.fda.gov/NewsEvents/ Newsroom/PressAnnouncements/2008/ucm116942.htm. Accessed April 11, 2016.
77. Olson TC, Bongartz T, Crowson CS, et al. Histoplasmosis infection in patients with rheumatoid arthritis, 1998-2009. BMC Infect Dis 2011;11:145.
78. Hage CA, Bowyer S, Tarvin SE, et al. Recognition, diagnosis, and treatment of histoplasmosis complicating tumor necrosis factor blocker therapy. Clin Infect Dis 2010;50:85–92.
79. Vergidis P, Avery RK, Wheat LJ, et al. Histoplasmosis complicating tumor necrosis factor-α blocker therapy: a retrospective analysis of 98 cases. Clin Infect Dis 2015;61:409–17.
80. Bergstrom L, Yocum DE, Ampel NM, et al. Increased risk of coccidioidomycosis in patients treated with tumor necrosis factor alpha antagonists. Arthritis Rheum 2004;50:1959–66.
81. Taroumian S, Knowles SL, Lisse JR, et al. Management of coccidioidomycosis in patients receiving biologic response modifiers or disease-modifying antirheumatic drugs. Arthritis Care Res (Hoboken) 2012;64:1903–9.

Malignancy and the Risks of Biologic Therapies

Current Status

Raphaèle Seror, MD, PhD[a,b,*], Xavier Mariette, MD, PhD[a,b]

KEYWORDS

- Skin cancer • Anti-TNF/TNF inhibitors • Biologic therapies • Lymphoma
- Abatacept • Rituximab • Tocilizumab

KEY POINTS

- The risk of cancer with anti–tumor necrosis factor (anti-TNF) has been extensively studied and the data are reassuring, showing no evidence overall of an increased risk of cancer.
- It is highly probable that anti-TNF is associated with an increased risk of nonmelanoma skin cancers, but possibly no different from that of other classic disease-modifying antirheumatic drugs.
- The risk of lymphoma does not seem to be increased with anti-TNF, but more data are required to analyze a possible dose effect and differential risk depending on the mechanism of action.
- Regarding other biologics, data are too few to draw any firm conclusion, although rituximab has reassuring data from its hematologic indications.

INTRODUCTION

Analyzing the risk of malignancy in rheumatic diseases is a complex situation. The occurrence of cancer in patients with rheumatic disease is common, as in the general population. At the age of 55 years, the typical age of rheumatoid arthritis (RA), about 20% of patients will be diagnosed with cancer during their remaining lifetimes. It represents the background risk applicable to all individuals and, and in most cases, the cancer has nothing to do with RA or its treatment. However, when analyzing this risk, some confounding factors have to be taken into account. In some cases, the cancer occurs as a result of factors also associated with the risk of developing rheumatic disease; for example, smoking and risk of RA. In a few cases, the malignancy could be

a INSERM U1184, Assistance Publique-Hôpitaux de Paris (AP-HP), Center of Research on Immunology of Viral and Autoimmune Diseases (IMVA), Université Paris-Sud, Le Kremlin Bicêtre, France; b Department of Rheumatology, Hôpitaux Universitaires Paris-Sud, Hôpital Bicêtre, 78 rue du Général Leclerc, Le Kremlin Bicêtre 94275, France
* Corresponding author. Department of Rheumatology, Hôpital Bicêtre, 78 rue du Général Leclerc, Le Kremlin Bicêtre 94275, France.
E-mail address: raphaele.se@gmail.com

Rheum Dis Clin N Am 43 (2017) 43–64
http://dx.doi.org/10.1016/j.rdc.2016.09.006
0889-857X/17/© 2016 Elsevier Inc. All rights reserved.

causally associated with the disease; for example, RA and lymphoma. In other cases, the treatment of the rheumatic disease could play a role in favoring cancer.

This article therefore analyzes the current knowledge on the risk of malignancy associated with biologics in rheumatic diseases but also provides some elements to better appraise it, and highlights some methodological issues to be kept in mind when evaluating the association between rheumatic diseases, treatments, and the risk of cancer.

HOW TO ASSESS THE RISK OF MALIGNANCY IN RHEUMATIC DISEASES?
Study Designs

Safety evaluation of new and existing drugs requires a careful assessment of the benefit/relative risk (RR). Malignancy represents a critical part of the safety profiles of biologics, because this risk if of low frequency, and may occur after long-term exposure.

Therefore, typical drug development programs, with limited sample size and follow-up, usually offer limited opportunity to assess this risk. To better appraise this risk, when analyzing literature, clinicians must keep in mind that estimating the risk of malignancies and also the risk of other rare severe side effects, may rely on a variety of studies designs. All these studies have different methodologies, and different advantages and weaknesses. Randomized controlled trials (RCTs) are intended to obtain an unbiased estimation of the efficacy and safety of a treatment under ideal conditions. Nevertheless, RCTs are not able to determine the potential effect of the treatment on the incidence of some rare adverse events because of the short duration of exposure to treatment and follow-up and limited patient numbers. To overcome these pitfalls, meta-analyses of RCTs help to obtain a larger sample size and therefore increase the power to analyze these risks, and long-term extension studies increase follow-up duration to identify risks associated with longer exposure to treatment, such as malignancies. Nevertheless, RCTs, their meta-analyses, and long-term extensions usually exclude patients with significant comorbidities, particularly patients with previous malignancies, who might be more prone to develop new cancers. Their results may not be able to be generalized to all treated patients in real-life settings. Therefore, observational designs are useful to analyze these risks in real-world settings. In contrast, on RCTs, observational studies offer the advantage of analyzing these risks in unselected large study populations with a longer follow-up. Nevertheless, their designs expose them to many other biases and particularly the difficulty of taking into account the impact of all potential confounders, known or unknown. Numerous study designs exist. Prospective cohort studies (including biologic registries) generally focused on 1 condition or on 1 drug or therapeutic class. These studies usually include more patients than RCTs and real-life patients (ie, with comorbid conditions). Such a design offers the advantage of having detailed data on the underlying disease, treatment, and comorbidities; it is important to take these elements into account because they are potential confounders in the estimation of risk. Nevertheless, these studies might still be underpowered to detect some rare risks. Another design relies on analysis of health insurance databases. These surveys usually have less information on the disease of interest and potential confounders, but have much more power and an incontestable representativeness.

Therefore, all the designs mentioned earlier give complementary information and are useful to analyze the risk of malignancies. Above all, it is the concordance between the results of all these different designs that allows confidence in the estimation of these risks.

Comparator Groups

When analyzing the risk of malignancy associated with a treatment, the choice of a comparator (reference) group is critical. The context of RCTs is the only one in which the comparator group has similar characteristics to the exposed group and is therefore comparable. Nevertheless, if this is true for the placebo-controlled phase of the trial, during the later phases and extension, the patients of the placebo arm are usually exposed to the drug. In observational studies, the choice of the comparator group is more challenging; to analyze the risk of a specific treatment correctly, the comparator should have the same baseline risk of malignancy as the exposed group.

If the general population is chosen for such analysis, the estimated risk also includes the risk of the underlying disease. In this case, the risk is usually expressed using the standardized incidence ratio (SIR). For studies conducted in only 1 country, it is best to use, when it exists, a database of cancers in the general population from the same country. This methodology is frequently used in Scandinavian studies. For multinational studies, 2 different general population databases are available for this type of comparison: the Surveillance, Epidemiology, and End Results (SEER) program of the National Cancer Institute, which provides information on cancer statistics among the US population (available from: www.seer.cancer.gov); and the GLOBOCAN (available from: www.globocan.iarc.fr), which provides contemporary estimates of the incidence, prevalence, and mortality from major types of cancer, at the national level, for 184 countries.[1] In rheumatic diseases, most multinational studies use SEER as the comparator, whereas it should be more logical to use GLOBOCAN.

To analyze of the risk of cancer associated with the use of biologics, the ideal comparator group should be patients having the same underlying disease and the same disease severity. This ideal control group most often does not exist and, usually, the control group for patients receiving biologics consists of patients receiving conventional disease-modifying antirheumatic drugs (DMARDs),[2] usually methotrexate. In this situation, the risk is expressed as either hazard ratio (HR), odds ratio (OR), or RR.

RISK OF CANCER IN RHEUMATIC DISEASES: IS THERE A ROLE OF THE UNDERLYING DISEASE?

The risk of cancer in rheumatic diseases has principally been studied in RA. It has been shown that patients with RA have an increased risk of developing some malignancies, particularly lymphoma,[3] leukemia, and lung cancer, compared with the general population but have a reduced risk of developing colorectal and breast cancer.[3–5]

Overall, the risk of cancer in RA is increased only marginally or not at all.[6]

The risk of cancer in patients with diseases other than RA is uncertain. The risk of solid malignancies, lymphomas, or leukemia does not seem to be increased in patients with ankylosing spondylitis (AS).[7,8] Also, patients with psoriatic arthritis (PsA) have a risk of cancer comparable with the risk in the general population, and possibly a modestly increased rate of lymphoma, as in patients with psoriasis.[7,9,10] In contrast, some older studies show a decreased risk of rectal cancer related to the use of nonsteroidal antiinflammatory drugs, and an increased risk of unspecified kidney cancer, in one study probably related to frequent radiographic pelvic examinations.[11] Patients with lupus and Sjögren syndrome have an increased risk of lymphoma.[4,12] Also, patients with systemic sclerosis have a 1.5-times to 5-times increased risk of malignant diseases. Both solid tumors and lymphoproliferative diseases may develop among them, but lung cancer was the most frequent type of cancer in most studies.[13]

RISK OF CANCER IN RHEUMATIC DISEASE: IS THERE A ROLE OF TREATMENT?

Taking all this information together, the relative roles of the underlying disease and of the treatments acting on the immune system, such as biologics, remain difficult to analyze. Some of these risks (eg, lymphoma) are at least partly driven by inflammation and disease activity.[14] Therefore, patients who are going to be treated with the most powerful immunosuppressant are also frequently the patients the most at risk of lymphoma. In contrast, a good control of disease activity by these powerful immunosuppressants should, with time, decrease the risk of lymphomas linked to activity of the disease.

First, because control populations are usually patients with conventional DMARDs, before analyzing the risk of malignancies associated with biologic therapies, it is necessary to know the risk of these treatments. No strong data suggest that conventional DMARDs, including methotrexate and sulfasalazine, alter the overall risk of cancer, except a possible increased risk of nonmelanoma skin cancer (NMSC) associated with methotrexate.[15,16] Even if some Epstein-Barr virus–associated lymphoma may occur on methotrexate,[17,18] overall, the risk of lymphoma does not seem to be increased with methotrexate,[19] except in 2 studies in Japan: in the NinJa cohort, use of methotrexate increased the risk of lymphoma: OR – 3.5 (2.0–6.3).[20] In another case-control study in Japan a higher dose of methotrexate was associated with a higher risk of lymphoma.[21] Concerning azathioprine and cyclosporine, there is some evidence of a possible increased risk of posttransplant lymphoproliferative disorders.[14,22]

Anti–tumor Necrosis Factor Alpha and Malignancies

Being the first to be approved, anti–tumor necrosis factor alpha (anti-TNF) inhibitors have been the most studied drugs. Five anti-TNFs are now approved for the treatment of RA and AS, some of them also being marketed for the treatment of PsA, cutaneous psoriasis, and inflammatory colitis. Infliximab, adalimumab, and the 2 most recent drugs, certolizumab and golimumab, are monoclonal antibodies directed against TNF, whereas etanercept is a fusion protein of human p75 soluble TNF receptor and human immunoglobulin G1. Most of the data come from the first 3 anti-TNFs developed (etanercept, adalimumab, and infliximab).

Risk of solid cancer

In 2006, in an important a publication from the *Journal of the American Medical Association*, the first meta-analyses of RCTs of adalimumab and infliximab in RA reported a significantly increased risk of cancer mainly because of an increased risk of lymphomas.[23] In this meta-analysis including 9 trials, 29 out of 3493 cancers (including 8 lymphomas) were reported in anti-TNF–treated patients versus 3 out of 1594 (no lymphoma) in the pooled placebo arms (**Table 1**). The RR of malignancy was estimated to be 3.3 (95% confidence interval [CI], 1.2–9.1) updated to 2.4 (95% CI, 1.2–4.8) a few months later with 2 additional trials. Nevertheless, this study has a major methodological issue, which is that incidence of cancers was analyzed by randomized patients and not by person-years at risk. Because the population was highly selected with a very low risk of cancer by history and because of baseline examinations, the observed risk of malignancy in the placebo group at inclusion was 12% of what was expected for the people of the same age and sex in the general population. With time, the risk of cancer tends to reach the risk of the general population. Because the follow-up is longer in the anti-TNF arm because of discontinuation for lack of efficacy in the placebo arm, the anti-TNF group may be disadvantaged. Later, an individual-data meta-analysis of etanercept RCTs in RA analyzed the risk of cancer in person-years, and showed a

Table 1
Meta-analyses and large observational studies assessing the risk of overall malignancies in anti–tumor necrosis factor patients compared with biologic-naive patients

	Indication	Number of Studies	Drugs	Risk of Overall Malignancies Risk (OR, RR, or HR) (95% CI)
Meta-analyses of RCTs				
Bongartz et al,[23] 2006	RA	7 9	Infliximab Adalimumab	OR = 3.29 (1.19–9.08) Revised: OR = 2.4 (1.2–4.8)
Bongartz et al,[24] 2009	RA	9	Etanercept	OR = 1.8 (0.8–4.3)
Leombruno et al,[31] 2009	RA	18	Infliximab Adalimumab Etanercept	Recommended doses: OR = 1.34 (95% CI, 0.75–2.39) High dose: OR = 2.49 (0.82–7.59) Including skin cancer and hematologic malignancies
Askling et al,[25] 2011	All inflammatory diseases	74	Infliximab Adalimumab Etanercept	HR = 0.99 (0.61–1.68) Excluding NMSC
Lopez-Olivo et al,[26] 2012	RA	63	Infliximab Adalimumab Etanercept Certolizumab Golimumab	OR = 1.31 (0.78–2.20) (20 trials) Solid tumors (excluding skin cancer and hematologic malignancies)
Thompson et al,[29] 2011	Early RA	6	Infliximab Adalimumab Etanercept	OR = 1.08 (0.50–2.32)
Le Blay et al,[40] 2012	RA	6	Certolizumab Golimumab	OR = 1.06 (0.39–2.85) Excluding NMSC
Liu et al,[30] 2014	RA	34	Infliximab Adalimumab Etanercept Certolizumab Golimumab	All doses: RR (ITT): 1.37 (0.87–2.17) High dose: RR (ITT): 2.39 (1.13–5.05) Approved dose: RR (ITT): 1.30 (0.80–2.14) Low dose: RR (ITT): 0.53 (0.16–1.80)

(continued on next page)

Table 1
(continued)

	Indication	Number of Studies	Drugs	Risk of Overall Malignancies Risk (OR, RR, or HR) (95% CI)
Michaud et al,[28] 2014	RA	44	Infliximab Adalimumab Etanercept Certolizumab Golimumab	OR = 1.29 (0.85–1.97)
Singh et al,[27] 2016	RA	79 Including 19 reporting cancer data	—	All anti-TNF = 9 trials OR = 1.21(0.63–2.38) All biologics: 16 trials OR = 1.07 (0.68–1.58)
Pooled Analyses of Observational Studies or Large Database				
Mariette et al,[32] 2011	RA, AS	29 studies of 12 registries	Infliximab Adalimumab Etanercept	0.95 (0.85–1.05)
Nyboe Andersen et al,[39] 2014	IBD	4 databases 4553 patients/56,146 patients	Infliximab Adalimumab Certolizumab	RR = 1.07 (0.85–1.36)
Haynes et al,[35] 2013	RA	Anti-TNF = 19,750 patients Not exposed = 9805 patients	Infliximab Adalimumab Etanercept	During exposure: HR = 0.80 (0.59–1.08) Until start of an alternative treatment: HR = 0.94 (0.79–1.12)
Wu et al,[37] 2014	RA	Anti-TNF = 4426 patients Not exposed = 17,704 patients	All anti-TNF	aHR: 0.63 (0.49–0.80) SIR = 0.83 (0.65, 1.04) Anti-TNF vs Taiwanese general population as reference
Harigai et al,[38] 2016	RA	Biologic exposed: 14,440 patients	Infliximab, etanercept, adalimumab, golimumab, tocilizumab, or abatacept	SIR = 0.75 (0.67–0.83) All biologics vs Japanese general population as reference

Abbreviations: aHR, adjusted hazard ratio; AS, ankylosing spondylitis; CI, confidence interval; IBD, inflammatory bowel disease; ITT, intention to treat.

nonsignificant but increased risk compared with controls (RR = 1.8; 95% CI, 0.8–4.3).[24] Nevertheless, all recent meta-analyses, one including 74 RCTs with the first 3 anti-TNFs in all indications,[25] and 3 including 63, 44, and 79 trials restricted to patients with RA, but including the more recent anti-TNF,[26–28] did not find any overall increased risk of malignancies, whatever the molecule (see **Table 1**). Similar results were found in early RA trials.[29] An additional meta-analysis that focused on the risk of breast cancer and overall malignancies suggested a possible increased risk of malignancies when anti-TNFs were prescribed at doses higher than the marketed doses,[30] but this was not found in other meta-analyses.[28,31]

Data from observational studies did not either show an overall increased risk of solid cancer. Among them, in a meta-analysis of all RA registries,[32] the pooled estimate for the risk of all-site malignancy from 7 studies was 0.95 (95% CI, 0.85–1.05). These analyses relied on the most recent update of the large registries at the time of analyses, including RABBIT (Rheumatoid Arthritis Observation of Biologic Therapy) (German), ARTIS (Antirheumatic Therapies in Sweden) (Sweden), BIOBADASER (Base de Datos de Productos Biológicos de la Sociedad Española de Reumatología), LOHREN (Lombardy Rheumatology Network), NDBRB (National Data Bank for Rheumatic Diseases), CORRONA (Consortium of Rheumatology Researchers of North America), and BSRBR registries.[33] Recent analysis of the DANBIO (Danish Nationwide Biologic) registry also found no increased risk in patients with AS treated with anti-TNF compared with biologic-naive patients (RR, 0.8; 95% CI, 0.7–1.0).[34] Also, analyses from health insurance databases, such as the US SABER (Safety Assessment of Biologic ThERapy) database,[35] confirm the absence of the overall increased risk of malignancies. This analysis included 29,555 patients with RA (19,750 taking an anti-TNF, 9805 taking a comparator drug). Although methodology varied widely between these studies, the relative risk of cancer among patients receiving TNF inhibitors was not increased compared with the patients treated with traditional DMARDs.[2,36] In addition, in 2 Asian studies, the health insurance database study in Taiwan[37] and the SECURE (SafEty of biologics in Clinical Use in Japanese patients with RhEumatoid arthritis) registry in Japan,[38] the latter including 14,440 patients with a follow-up of 49,320 patients-years, the risk of cancer was decreased compared with the general population: SIR = 0.83 (0.65, 1.04) and 0.75 (0.67–0.83), respectively. This decreased risk is probably the consequence of the selection of the patients who are eligible for anti-TNF treatment.

The analysis of the Danish registry in another important indication of anti-TNF, namely inflammatory bowel disease (IBD), confirmed that exposure to anti-TNF among patients with IBD was not associated with an increased risk of cancer, whatever the duration of exposition and the age at the initiation of the first anti-TNF.[39] Importantly, most of these data concern the 3 first marketed anti-TNFs, but the most recent studies derived from RCTs or observational studies with certolizumab[26,40] and golimumab lead to the same conclusions but with less power.[38]

Risk of skin cancer
Nonmelanoma skin cancer Regarding skin cancers, the situation is different (**Table 2**). The larger meta-analyses of 76 trials showed an increased risk of NMSC with an HR of 2.02 (95% CI, 1.11, 3.95).[25] However, other meta-analyses with fewer studies did not show any increased risk.[26,31,40] Long-term extension studies of RCTs of adalimumab also suggest an increased risk of NMSC.[41] In the meta-analysis of registries, results from 4 studies showed that patients treated with anti-TNF have a significantly increased risk of developing an NMSC, with an RR of 1.33 (95% CI, 1.06, 1.60).[32,42] However, analysis of the Danish registry found an increased risk of NMSC in patients with RA treated

Table 2
Studies analyzing the risk of nonmelanoma skin cancer and melanoma with anti-tumor necrosis factor

Study	Indication	Number of Studies	Drugs	Risk of Nonmelanoma Skin Cancer Risk (OR, RR, or HR) (95% CI)	Risk of Melanoma Risk (OR, RR, or HR) (95% CI)
Meta-analyses of Randomized Controlled Trials					
Leombruno et al,[31] 2009	RA, AS	18	Infliximab Adalimumab Etanercept	Recommended dose OR = 1.27 (0.67–2.42) High dose 0.93 (0.27–3.16)	—
Askling et al,[25] 2011	All	74	Infliximab Adalimumab Etanercept	HR = 2.02 (1.11–3.95)	—
Lopez-Olivo et al,[26] 2012	RA	63	Infliximab Adalimumab Etanercept Certolizumab Golimumab	OR = 1.37 (0.59–3.19) 12 studies	OR = 1.08 (0.11–10.21) 3 studies
Le Blay et al,[40] 2012	RA	6	Certolizumab Golimumab	OR = 0.69 (95% CI, 0.23–2.11)	—
Long-term Extension of RCTs					
Burmester et al,[41] 2013	RA AS PsA Ps CD	71 (23 458 patients)	Adalimumab	In RA: SIR = 1.39 (1.19–1.60) In Ps: SIR = 1.76 (1.26–2.39) In CD: SIR = 2.29 (1.44–4.47) Not increased in patients with AS and PsA Anti-TNF vs general population (SEER as reference)	In RA: SIR = 1.5 (0.84–2.47) In Ps: SIR = 4.37 (1.89–8.61) Anti-TNF vs general population (SEER as reference)
Pooled Analyses of Observational Studies					
Mariette et al,[32] 2011	RA	29 studies of 12 registries	Infliximab Adalimumab Etanercept	RR: 1.33 (95% CI, 1.06, 1.60)	RR: 1.79 (0.92–2.67)

Study	Disease	Biologic	Number of Patients		
Nyboe Andersen et al,[39] 2014	IBD	Infliximab Adalimumab Certolizumab	4 databases Anti-TNF:4553 patients Not exposed: 56,146	—	RR: 1.31 (0.63-2.74) Adjusted for azathioprine use
Observational Studies			Number of Patients		
Mercer et al,[48] 2012, BSRBR	RA	—	Anti-TNF = 11,881 Not exposed = 3629	Overall HR = 0.95 (0.53-1.71) Basal cell cancer HR = 1.2 (0.8-1.7) Squamous cell cancer HR = 1.8 (0.6-5.4) Anti-TNF vs biologic naive	—
Haynes et al,[35] 2013, SABER	RA	Infliximab Adalimumab Etanercept	Anti-TNF = 19,750 Not exposed = 9805	During exposure: HR = 0.83 (0.49-1.42) Until start of an alternative treatment: HR = 1.07 (0.79-1.46)	—
Dreyer et al,[43] 2013, DANBIO	RA AS PsA	—	Anti-TNF = 5345 Not exposed = 4351	HR = 1.10 (0.69-1.76) Anti-TNF vs biologic naive SIR = 1.92 (1.42-2.59) Anti-TNF vs general population	HR = 1.54 (0.37-6.34) Anti-TNF vs biologic naive SIR = 1.57 (0.70-3.49) Anti-TNF vs general population
Raaschou et al,[47] 2013, ARTIS	RA	—	Anti-TNF = 10,878 Not exposed = 42,198	—	Invasive melanoma HR = 1.2 (0.9-1.5) Biologic naive vs Swedish general population HR = 1.5 (1.0-2.2) Anti-TNF vs biologic naive In situ melanoma HR = 1.2 (0.9-1.7) Biologic naive vs Swedish general population HR = 1.1 (0.5-2.1) Anti-TNF vs biologic naive

(continued on next page)

Table 2
(continued)

Study	Indication	Number of Studies	Drugs	Risk of Nonmelanoma Skin Cancer Risk (OR, RR, or HR) (95% CI)	Risk of Melanoma Risk (OR, RR, or HR) (95% CI)
Raaschou et al,[44] 2016, ARTIS	RA	Anti-TNF (n = 12,558) Not exposed (n = 46,409)	—	Basal cell cancer HR = 1.22 (1.07–1.41) Biologic naive vs Swedish general population HR = 1.14 (0.98–1.33) Anti-TNF vs biologic naive Squamous cell cancer HR = 1.88 (1.74–2.03) Biologic naive vs Swedish general population HR = 1.30 (1.10–1.55) Anti-TNF vs biologic naive	—
Wu et al,[37] 2014	RA	Anti-TNF = 4426 Not exposed = 17,704	All anti-TNF	SIR = 2.05 (0.66–4.79) Anti-TNF vs Taiwanese general population as reference	—
Harigai et al,[38] 2016, SECURE database	RA	Biologic exposed: 14,440	Infliximab Etanercept Adalimumab Golimumab Tocilizumab Abatacept	All skin cancer SIR = 1.190 (0.340–2.210) All biologics vs Japanese general population as reference	—

with anti-TNF only compared with the general population, with a SIR estimated at 1.92 (95% CI, 1.4–2.6), which was the same as the increased risk found in patients treated with conventional DMARDs (SIR = 1.76; 95% CI, 1.3–2.5), without any difference between anti-TNF and conventional DMARDs.[43] These results are in line with recent data showing that methotrexate use is associated with an increased risk of a second NMSC (in patients with previous NMSC), similar to the risk associated with anti-TNF use particularly when used with methotrexate for RA.[16] Nevertheless, the results of the ARTIS registry confirm the increased risk of NMSC in patients with RA, showing an increased risk of basal cell cancer (HR = 1.22; 95% CI, 1.07–1.41) in biologic-naive patients with RA compared with the general population but no additional significant increase in risk in anti-TNF–treated patients (HR = 1.14 [0.98–1.33]; 236 vs 1587 events) compared with biologic-naive patients. In contrast, for squamous cell cancer skin cancer, the HR was 1.88 (1.74–2.03) comparing biologic-naive patients with RA with the general population, and 1.30 (1.10–1.55; 191 vs 847 events) comparing TNF inhibitors with biologic-naive patients, showing an additional risk associated with anti-TNF use.[44]

Melanoma Regarding the risk of melanoma, the literature is even more controversial (see **Table 2**). The question of melanoma and anti-TNF is pertinent because TNF infusions have been used to treat some locally advanced melanoma.[45,46] Thus there was a theoretic risk that anti-TNF could increase the risk of occurrence of melanoma. The meta-analysis of the registries found an increased, but not significant, risk of developing melanoma in patients treated with anti-TNF, because the pooled estimate from 2 studies was 1.79 (95% CI, 0.92–2.67).[32] Data from the Swedish registry, ARTIS, showed a significant increased risk of invasive melanoma (but not in situ melanoma) in patients treated with anti-TNF compared with patients treated by conventional DMARDs (HR = 1.5; 95% CI, 1.0–2.2).[47] Nevertheless, this risk remains controversial.[16,25,32,43,47] In addition, a combined analysis of 11 European registries did not find any increased risk of melanoma with anti-TNF.[49]

Risk of lymphoma

Compared with the general population, patients with RA are at an increased risk of lymphoma, but not AS. This risk is estimated at around 2 to 3 times that of the general population, and is slightly higher in Asiatic populations.[3,4,12,37,38] This risk of lymphoma in RA is at least partly driven by inflammation and disease activity.[14] Thus, observational studies are exposed to a major indication bias, because patients treated with biologics are those with longer disease duration and higher disease activity; that is, they are at higher risk of developing lymphoma. In contrast, a good control of disease activity by these powerful immunosuppressive drugs should, with time, decrease the risk of lymphomas linked to activity of the disease. Nevertheless, most observational studies could not account for activity over the duration of the disease. To deal with the complicated issue of lymphoma and biologics in rheumatic diseases, note that lymphoma caused by disease activity and by immunosuppression are frequently of different subtypes. Likewise, activity of the disease is associated with activated B-cell and diffuse large B-cell lymphoma in RA and mucosa-associated lymphoid tissue lymphoma in Sjögren syndrome, whereas immunosuppression-associated lymphomas have characteristics of posttransplant lymphoproliferative disease frequently associated with lymphoma. Thus, a careful examination of the types of lymphoma is useful but rarely done.

In meta-analyses of RCTs that are not exposed to such bias, no increased risk of lymphoma has been observed (**Table 3**), but the number of events is low, the duration of exposition is limited, and thus they are usually underpowered.[26,50]

Table 3
Studies analyzing the risk of lymphoma with anti–tumor necrosis factor

Study	Indication	Number of Studies	Drugs	Risk of Lymphoma Compared with RA Controls Risk (OR, RR, o⁻ HR) (95% CI)	Risk of Lymphoma Compared with General Population SIR (95% CI)
Meta-analyses of Randomized Controlled Trials					
Leombruno et al,[31] 2009	RA	18	Infliximab Adalimumab Etanercept	Standard doses OR = 1.26 (0.52–3.06) High doses: OR = 1.14 (0.28–4.61)	—
Lopez-Olivo et al,[26] 2012	RA	63	Infliximab Adalimumab Etanercept Certolizumab Golimumab	2.14 (0.55–8.38) 10 studies	—
Long-term Extension Studies					
Weinblatt et al,[51] 2011	RA	9	Etanercept	—	Early RA SIR = 5.8 (2.33–11.94) Long-standing RA SIR = 4.1 (1.63–8.37) SEER as reference
Bykerk et al,[53] 2015	RA	10	Certolizumab	—	S R = 2.72 (0.88–6.34) GLOBOCAN as reference S R = 1.81 (0.59–4.23) SEER database as reference
Burmester et al,[41] 2013	RA AS PsA	71 (23,458 patients)	Adalimumab	—	SIR = 2.74 (CI, 1.83–3.93) SEER as reference
Kay et al,[52] 2015	RA AS PsA	6	Golimumab	—	Dose of 100 mg monthly SIR = 6.69 (2.45–14.56) Dose of 50 mg monthly SIR = 1.71 (0.04–9.55) SEER as reference

Pooled Analyses of Observational Studies

Mariette et al,[32] 2011	RA and AS	29 studies of 12 registries	Infliximab Adalimumab Etanercept	RR: 1.11 (0.70–1.51)	RR: 2.55 (1.93–3.17)
Nyboe Andersen et al,[39] 2014	IBD	4 databases Anti-TNF: 4553 patients Not exposed: 56,146	Infliximab Adalimumab Certolizumab	All hematologic malignancies: RR = 1.36 (0.67–2.76) RR = 0.90 (0.42–1.91) adjusted for azathioprine use	—
Observational Studies[a]					
Mariette et al,[55] 2010 (RATIO)	All indications	38 cases of lymphoma	Infliximab Adalimumab Etanercept	Etanercept as reference Infliximab: OR = 4.73 (1.27–17.65) Adalimumab: OR = 4.12 (1.36–12.49)	Overall: SIR = 2.4 (1.7–3.2) Infliximab or adalimumab: SIR = 3.7 (2.6–5.3) Etanercept: SIR = 0.9 (0.4–1.8)
Haynes et al,[35] 2013	RA	Anti-TNF: 19,750 Not exposed: 9805	Infliximab Adalimumab Etanercept	During exposure: HR = 0.83 (0.33–2.05) Until start of an alternative treatment: HR = 1.25 (0.71–2.20)	—
Wu et al,[37] 2014	RA	Anti-TNF: 4426 Not exposed: 17,704	All anti-TNF	—	SIR = 6.13 (3.26, 10.49) Taiwanese general population as reference
Harigai et al,[38] 2016	RA	Biologic exposed: 14,440	Infliximab, etanercept, adalimumab, golimumab, tocilizumab, or abatacept	—	SIR = 6.18 (4.81–7.64) All biologics vs Japanese general population as reference Infliximab: IR = 3.38; (2.57–4.38) Etanercept: IR = 1.30 (0.87–1.87)

[a] Published after the 2011 meta-analysis of Mariette and colleagues,[32] or providing additional information.

In long-term extension studies, the incidence of lymphoma was increased in patients with RA treated with anti-TNF, usually within the range expected in RA without anti-TNF therapy.[41,51–53] Also, patients treated with higher dose of golimumab (100 mg monthly) might be at greater risk of lymphoma than is expected in patients with RA (SIR = 14.13 [1.71–51.03] during the placebo-controlled phase and 6.69 [2.45–14.56] including the long-term extension phase).[52,54] In contrast, at a 50-mg monthly dosage, the SIR was 0.00 (0.00–32.66) during the placebo-controlled phase and 1.71 (0.04–9.55) including the long-term extension phase. Thus, even being cautious because the CI is wide, it is possible that, at high doses, anti-TNF could have a deleterious effect concerning the risk of lymphoma.

Observational studies and their meta-analysis showed an expected increased risk of lymphoma compared with the general population, with an SIR of 2.55 (95% CI, 1.93–3.17), but no increased risk compared with RA treated with conventional DMARDs, with a pooled estimate for the risk of lymphoma of 1.11 (95% CI, 0.70–1.51).[32] However, some studies suggest that the risk might be different according to the mechanism of action, with a possible lower risk with etanercept,[38,55,56] but these data need to be confirmed. In the French observatory RATIO, 38 cases were collected in 3 years and compared with the general population and a cohort of RA treated with anti-TNF but having no lymphoma.[55] The overall risk of lymphoma in this population of patients with RA treated with the 2 monoclonal antibodies compared with that of the general population was increased as expected in a population of patients with severe RA (SIR = 3.7; 95% CI, 2.6–5.3). However, this higher risk compared with the general population was not found for etanercept (SIR = 0.9; 95% CI, 0.4–1.8). Likewise, in the nationwide Japanese SECURE registry, there was an increased risk of lymphoma compared with the general population (SIR = 6.18; 95% CI, 4.81–7.64) and the risk was greater with infliximab than with etanercept (incidence rate = 3.38, 95% CI, 2.57–4.38; and incidence rate = 1.30, 95% CI, 0.87–1.87, respectively; P<6.6 10–4).[38] In addition, a possible decreased risk of lymphoma in patients treated with etanercept, compared with patients treated (adjusted hazard ratio [aHR] [95% CIs], 0.51 [0.28, 0.95]) with conventional DMARDs has been found in the British registry.[56] However, the lymphoma risk with the 2 monoclonal antibodies was not reported.

Risk of recurrent cancer

Because of their mechanisms of action, anti-TNFs are contraindicated in patients with recent malignancies (<5 years). Nevertheless, even if alternative therapies are available in RA, in other inflammatory disorders, such as and PsA, anti-TNFs remain the key and sometimes the only available biologics. Therefore, another important issue is how to treat patient with previous malignancy and what is the risk of recurrent malignancies. In the Swedish registry ARTIS, comparison of the outcomes of patients with previous breast cancer showed a difference between patients treated with anti-TNFs and those treated with conventional DMARDs (aHRs [95% CIs], 1.1 [0.4, 2.8]) regarding the risk of recurrence.[57] Two other publications have examined the risk of developing further malignancy in patients with previous malignancy before receiving treatment with anti-TNF. In RABBIT, the incidence rate ratio (IRR) for patients treated with anti-TNF compared with DMARD was 1.4 (95% CI, 0.5–5.5; P = .63).[58] In the BSRBR, the adjusted IRR in patients with a previous malignancy was 0.45 (95% CI, 0.09–2.17; propensity score adjusted).[59] The differences between the studies may reflect the longer time from primary cancer to the initiation of anti-TNF in BSRBR compared with RABBIT (median 8.5 vs 5 years).[60] Censoring after the first incident of malignancy did not affect the results. In the meta-analysis of registries, a pooled analysis resulted in an overall risk estimate of 0.62 (95% CI, 0.04–1.20).[32] Nevertheless, even if data from the UK and

German registries are reassuring, they rely on small numbers of patients.[57–59] Also in the analysis from RABBIT, it was reported that 14 out of the 15 cancers were true recurrences of the previous cancer. Although less is known from patients with recent malignancy, data for patients with IBDs seem reassuring. Nevertheless, data from the RABBIT registry require caution, and suggest that such indications have to be case-by-case joint decisions taken with the patient and the oncologist.[61]

Another frequent situation is the human papilloma virus infection and the risk of cervical malignancies. In the BSRBR and DANBIO registries, 190 and 327 women with histories of premalignant cervix lesions treated with anti-TNF were compared with 48 and 598 women treated with conventional DMARDs with no increased risk of cervical cancer.[62,63] However, it is possible that conventional DMARDs might also be at risk of recurrence of cervical lesions. In the more recent data from the ARTIS registry, results are more worrisome. In the biologic-naive patients with RA, there were significantly higher rates of cervical intraepithelial neoplasia (CIN) 1 (HR, 1.53; 95% CI, 1.23–1.89) and CIN 2+ (HR, 1.39; 95% CI, 1.16–1.66) but not of invasive cancer (HR 1.09, 95% CI 0.71–1.65 for the overall population; and HR 0.78, 95% CI 0.36–1.70), when restricting to individuals with a history of a normal screening test before start of follow-up. In the anti-TNF cohort, there was no statistically significant difference in risk for CIN 1 (HR, 1.23; 95% CI, 0.87–1.74), but a higher rate of CIN 2+ (HR, 1.36; 95% CI, 1.01–1.82) and a doubled risk of invasive cervical cancer in the anti-TNF cohort (HR, 2.10; 95% CI, 1.04–4.23). Even when restricting the analysis to individuals with a normal screening test as the last screening before start of follow-up, 10 cases of invasive cervical cancer were observed, corresponding with an HR of 3.77 (95% CI, 1.35–10.48).[64]

Pediatric rheumatology
Few data are available from pediatric rheumatology. Nevertheless, the overall incidence of malignancy for pediatric patients seems to be higher compared with the aged-matched pediatric population. This increase in overall reporting rate seems to consistently be because of the increase in reports of lymphoma (mainly Hodgkin), with higher incidence rates than those reported in the general population,[65,66] and this may also be at least partly linked to the risk of the underlying disease.[67]

Other Biologics and Malignancies

Other biologics have been much less studied (**Table 4**). Experience from hematologic indications with rituximab did not reveal major risks; data in inflammatory disorders are sparse. Most of the data rely on RCTs, meta-analyses, and long-term extension studies. These biologics have been marketed only recently and data from registries are still underpowered to allow firm conclusions.

Meta-analyses and long-term extensions studies
In the meta-analysis including all biologics, no overall increased risk of malignancies has been observed with any of the biologics,[26] but CIs are wide because only 4 studies have been included for each of the biologics other than anti-TNF.

The long-term safety report for the clinical development program of rituximab included 3595 patients followed up to 11 years (14,816 patient-years), and did not indicate an increased risk of malignancy for patients receiving rituximab with RA (SIR, 1.07; 95% CI, 0.88–1.29) compared with the general US population (SEER database) and compared with published data in adults with RA.[68]

Comparison of 4134 patients with RA treated with abatacept included in 7 trials of the clinical development program and 41,529 conventional DMARD-treated patients

Table 4
Risk of malignancies associated with biologics other than anti-tumor necrosis factor: randomized controlled trials and long-term extension studies data

Study	Indication	Number of Studies	Drugs	Risk of Overall Malignancies	Risk of Lymphoma	Risk of Melanoma	Risk of Nonmelanoma Skin Cancer
Meta-analyses of Randomized Controlled Trials				Compared with RA Controls			
Lopez-Olivo et al,[26] 2012	RA	63	All anti-TNF Abatacept Rituximab Tocilizumab	Abatacept (4 trials) OR = 0.82 (0.22–3.01) Rituximab (4 trials) OR = 2.28 (0.72–7.25) Tocilizumab (4 trials) OR = 2.22 (0.79–6.20) Solid tumors (excluding skin cancer and hematologic malignancies)	Abatacept (1 trial) OR = 4.51 (0.07–285.89) Tocilizumab (1 trial) OR = 0.05 (0.00–3.19)	No trial	Abatacept (3 trials) OR = 0.54 (0.13–2.31) Tocilizumab (2 trials) OR = 0.22 (0.02–2.44)
Singh et al,[27] 2016	RA	79	—	Non-anti-TNF biologic = OR 0.99 (0.58–1.78 (7 trials)	—	—	—
Long-term extension studies		Number of patients		Compared with General Population			
Van Vollenhoven et al,[68] 2015	RA	11 studies: 3595	Rituximab	SIR: 1.07 (0.88–1.29) SEER as reference	—	—	—
Weinblatt et al,[70] 2013	RA	7 studies: 4134	Abatacept	SIR: 0.99 (0.80, 1.22) SEER as reference	SIR: 2.49 (1.14, 4.73) SEER as reference	—	—
Rubbert-Roth et al,[72] 2016	RA	4009	Tocilizumab	SIR: 1.36 (1.01–1.80) SEER as reference SIR: 1.81 (1.44–2.23) GLOBOCAN as reference	Non-Hodgkin lymphoma SIR = 3.93 (1.07–10.18) SEER as reference	—	—
Yamamoto et al,[73] 2015	RA	5573	Tocilizumab	SIR: 0.79 (0.66–0.95) Japanese general population as reference	SIR: 3.13 (1.82–5.39) Japanese general population as reference	—	All skin cancer SIR: 1.44 (0.54–3.84)

with RA from the 5 observational cohorts revealed no increased risk of malignancies and lymphoma.[69] Analysis of long-term extension of 8 clinical trials of intravenous abatacept revealed no increased risk of overall malignancies (SIR = 0.99; 95% CI, 0.80, 1.22) and a risk of lymphoma within the usual range for patients with RA (9 events: SIR = 2.49; 95% CI, 1.14, 4.73).[70]

In combined analysis and long-term extension of tocilizumab trials, including 4009 exposed patients and 4199 controls, even if the first report did not reveal an increased risk of overall malignancies (SIR = 0.80; 95% CI, 0.78, 0.82),[71] the most recent updated data showed an SIR for all malignancies, excluding NMSC, of 1.36 (1.01–1.80) compared with the SEER database and 1.81 (1.44–2.23) compared with GLOBOCAN, suggesting an increased risk of malignancies.[72] In a Japanese study including 5573 patients who initiated intravenous tociluzumab, the proportion of malignancy during follow-up was 2.24% (0.83/100 patient-years), and the SIR was 0.79 (95% CI, 0.66–0.95). In this study, 13 lymphomas were observed with an SIR of 3.13 (95% CI, 1.82–5.39), taking the Japanese population as the reference.[73]

Registry data

More recent data from the CORRONA registry compared 1566 patients treated with methotrexate with those treated with biologics (3761 TNF antagonists, 408 abatacept, and 167 rituximab), and revealed no increased risk of cancer with abatacept (HR, 1.55; 95% CI, 0.40–5.97) or rituximab (HR, 0.42; 95% CI, 0.07–2.60). However, this study found an increased risk of cancer with methotrexate compared with anti-TNF (HR, 0.29; 95% CI, 0.05–0.65, in favor of anti-TNF). Nevertheless, the risk of NMSC seemed to be increased (HR, 15.3; 95% CI, 2.05–114) in abatacept-treated patients.

Regarding the risk of recurrent malignancies with biologics other than anti-TNF, recent data from the RABBIT registry revealed no major increased risk, but there were very few data. Of note, a low rate of recurrence has been observed in patients treated with rituximab, for which the risk was the same as for patients treated with conventional DMARDs. This finding is strengthened by the fact that the median time between prior solid malignancy and start of treatment was shorter in patients receiving rituximab than in all other treatments (median time 3.3 years compared with 5.2–6.8 years).[60]

SUMMARY

Fifteen years after coming on the market, the risk of cancer with anti-TNFs (particularly infliximab, adalimumab, and etanercept) has been largely studied and the data are reassuring. In spite of a concern in 2006, more recent meta-analyses of RCTs did not reveal any increased overall risk of cancer. However, the follow-up of these RCTs is short and the patients were selected. Observational studies did not find an increased risk either. However, it can also be argued that there is an indication bias in observational studies, meaning that the patients who are more at risk of cancer (previous cancer, premalignant lesions) were not treated with anti-TNFs. Thus, in these studies, because of this indication bias, a decreased risk of cancer could have been expected with anti-TNFs.[74] However, this has been observed in 2 Asian studies, the health insurance database study in Taiwan[37] and the SECURE registry in Japan.[38] In this context, new observational studies in patients with previous cancer will be important. It is probable that anti-TNFs are associated with an increased risk of NMSCs, but possibly not different from that of methotrexate or other immunosuppressive therapies. Also, even if up to now the overall risk of lymphoma does not seem to be increased, it is still necessary to remain cautious and particularly to have more data on a possible dose effect and on a possible differential risk depending on the mechanism of action. Regarding other biologics, data for rituximab are reassuring even in patients with recent malignancies and this treatment must be preferred in cases of previous malignancy. Until now, there is no known concern with the other biologics but data are too few to draw any firm conclusion.

REFERENCES

1. Ferlay J, Soerjomataram I, Dikshit R, et al. Cancer incidence and mortality worldwide: sources, methods and major patterns in GLOBOCAN 2012. Int J Cancer 2015;136:E359–86.
2. Solomon DH, Mercer E, Kavanaugh A. Observational studies on the risk of cancer associated with tumor necrosis factor inhibitors in rheumatoid arthritis: a review of their methodologies and results. Arthritis Rheum 2012;64:21–32.
3. Simon TA, Thompson A, Gandhi KK, et al. Incidence of malignancy in adult patients with rheumatoid arthritis: a meta-analysis. Arthritis Res Ther 2015;17:212.
4. Zintzaras E, Voulgarelis M, Moutsopoulos HM. The risk of lymphoma development in autoimmune diseases: a meta-analysis. Arch Intern Med 2005;165:2337–44.
5. Abasolo L, Judez E, Descalzo MA, et al. Cancer in rheumatoid arthritis: occurrence, mortality, and associated factors in a south European population. Semin Arthritis Rheum 2008;37:388–97.
6. Askling J. Malignancy and rheumatoid arthritis. Curr Rheumatol Rep 2007;9: 421–6.
7. Hellgren K, Smedby KE, Backlin C, et al. Ankylosing spondylitis, psoriatic arthritis, and risk of malignant lymphoma: a cohort study based on nationwide prospectively recorded data from Sweden. Arthritis Rheumatol 2014;66:1282–90.
8. Askling J, Klareskog L, Blomqvist P, et al. Risk for malignant lymphoma in ankylosing spondylitis: a nationwide Swedish case-control study. Ann Rheum Dis 2006;65:1184–7.
9. Gelfand JM, Shin DB, Neimann AL, et al. The risk of lymphoma in patients with psoriasis. J Invest Dermatol 2006;126:2194–201.
10. Carmona L, Abasolo L, Descalzo MA, et al. Cancer in patients with rheumatic diseases exposed to TNF antagonists. Semin Arthritis Rheum 2011;41:71–80.
11. Feltelius N, Ekbom A, Blomqvist P. Cancer incidence among patients with ankylosing spondylitis in Sweden 1965-95: a population based cohort study. Ann Rheum Dis 2003;62:1185–8.
12. Smedby KE, Hjalgrim H, Askling J, et al. Autoimmune and chronic inflammatory disorders and risk of non-Hodgkin lymphoma by subtype. J Natl Cancer Inst 2006;98:51–60.
13. Szekanecz E, Szamosi S, Horvath A, et al. Malignancies associated with systemic sclerosis. Autoimmun Rev 2012;11:852–5.
14. Baecklund E, Iliadou A, Askling J, et al. Association of chronic inflammation, not its treatment, with increased lymphoma risk in rheumatoid arthritis. Arthritis Rheum 2006;54:692–701.
15. Asten P, Barrett J, Symmons D. Risk of developing certain malignancies is related to duration of immunosuppressive drug exposure in patients with rheumatic diseases. J Rheumatol 1999;26:1705–14.
16. Scott FI, Mamtani R, Brensinger CM, et al. Risk of nonmelanoma skin cancer associated with the use of immunosuppressant and biologic agents in patients with a history of autoimmune disease and nonmelanoma skin cancer. JAMA Dermatol 2016;152(2):164–72.

17. Salloum E, Cooper DL, Howe G, et al. Spontaneous regression of lymphoproliferative disorders in patients treated with methotrexate for rheumatoid arthritis and other rheumatic diseases. J Clin Oncol 1996;14:1943–9.

18. Kamel OW, van de Rijn M, Weiss LM, et al. Brief report: reversible lymphomas associated with Epstein-Barr virus occurring during methotrexate therapy for rheumatoid arthritis and dermatomyositis. N Engl J Med 1993;328:1317–21.

19. Mariette X, Cazals-Hatem D, Warszawki J, et al. Lymphomas in rheumatoid arthritis patients treated with methotrexate: a 3-year prospective study in France. Blood 2002;99:3909–15.

20. Yamada T, Nakajima A, Inoue E, et al. Incidence of malignancy in Japanese patients with rheumatoid arthritis. Rheumatol Int 2011;31:1487–92.

21. Kameda T, Dobashi H, Miyatake N, et al. Association of higher methotrexate dose with lymphoproliferative disease onset in rheumatoid arthritis patients. Arthritis Care Res (Hoboken) 2014;66:1302–9.

22. Beaugerie L, Brousse N, Bouvier AM, et al. Lymphoproliferative disorders in patients receiving thiopurines for inflammatory bowel disease: a prospective observational cohort study. Lancet 2009;374:1617–25.

23. Bongartz T, Sutton AJ, Sweeting MJ, et al. Anti-TNF antibody therapy in rheumatoid arthritis and the risk of serious infections and malignancies: systematic review and meta-analysis of rare harmful effects in randomized controlled trials. JAMA 2006;295:2275–85.

24. Bongartz T, Warren FC, Mines D, et al. Etanercept therapy in rheumatoid arthritis and the risk of malignancies: a systematic review and individual patient data meta-analysis of randomised controlled trials. Ann Rheum Dis 2009;68:1177–83.

25. Askling J, Fahrbach K, Nordstrom B, et al. Cancer risk with tumor necrosis factor alpha (TNF) inhibitors: meta-analysis of randomized controlled trials of adalimumab, etanercept, and infliximab using patient level data. Pharmacoepidemiol Drug Saf 2011;20:119–30.

26. Lopez-Olivo MA, Tayar JH, Martinez-Lopez JA, et al. Risk of malignancies in patients with rheumatoid arthritis treated with biologic therapy: a meta-analysis. JAMA 2012;308:898–908.

27. Singh JA, Hossain A, Tanjong Ghogomu E, et al. Biologics or tofacitinib for rheumatoid arthritis in incomplete responders to methotrexate or other traditional disease-modifying anti-rheumatic drugs: a systematic review and network meta-analysis. Cochrane Database Syst Rev 2016;(5):CD012183.

28. Michaud TL, Rho YH, Shamliyan T, et al. The comparative safety of tumor necrosis factor inhibitors in rheumatoid arthritis: a meta-analysis update of 44 trials. Am J Med 2014;127:1208–32.

29. Thompson AE, Rieder SW, Pope JE. Tumor necrosis factor therapy and the risk of serious infection and malignancy in patients with early rheumatoid arthritis: a meta-analysis of randomized controlled trials. Arthritis Rheum 2011;63:1479–85.

30. Liu Y, Fan W, Chen H, et al. Risk of breast cancer and total malignancies in rheumatoid arthritis patients undergoing TNF-alpha antagonist therapy: a meta-analysis of randomized control trials. Asian Pac J Cancer Prev 2014;15:3403–10.

31. Leombruno JP, Einarson TR, Keystone EC. The safety of anti-tumour necrosis factor treatments in rheumatoid arthritis: meta and exposure-adjusted pooled analyses of serious adverse events. Ann Rheum Dis 2009;68:1136–45.

32. Mariette X, Matucci-Cerinic M, Pavelka K, et al. Malignancies associated with tumour necrosis factor inhibitors in registries and prospective observational studies: a systematic review and meta-analysis. Ann Rheum Dis 2011;70:1895–904.

33. Mercer LK, Lunt M, Low AL, et al. Risk of solid cancer in patients exposed to anti-tumour necrosis factor therapy: results from the British Society for Rheumatology Biologics Register for Rheumatoid Arthritis. Ann Rheum Dis 2015;74:1087–93.

34. Hellgren K, Dreyer L, Arkema EV, et al. Cancer risk in patients with spondyloarthritis treated with TNF inhibitors: a collaborative study from the ARTIS and DANBIO registers. Ann Rheum Dis 2016. http://dx.doi.org/10.1136/annrheumdis-2016-209270. [pii:annrheumdis-2016-209270].

35. Haynes K, Beukelman T, Curtis JR, et al. Tumor necrosis factor alpha inhibitor therapy and cancer risk in chronic immune-mediated diseases. Arthritis Rheum 2013;65:48–58.

36. Askling J, Berglind N, Franzen S, et al. How comparable are rates of malignancies in patients with rheumatoid arthritis across the world? A comparison of cancer rates, and means to optimise their comparability, in five RA registries. Ann Rheum Dis 2016;75(10):1789–96.

37. Wu CY, Chen DY, Shen JL, et al. The risk of cancer in patients with rheumatoid arthritis taking tumor necrosis factor antagonists: a nationwide cohort study. Arthritis Res Ther 2014;16:449.

38. Harigai M, Nanki T, Koike R, et al. Risk for malignancy in rheumatoid arthritis patients treated with biological disease-modifying antirheumatic drugs compared to the general population: a nationwide cohort study in Japan. Mod Rheumatol 2016;26(5):642–50.

39. Nyboe Andersen N, Pasternak B, Basit S, et al. Association between tumor necrosis factor-alpha antagonists and risk of cancer in patients with inflammatory bowel disease. Jama 2014;311:2406–13.

40. Le Blay P, Mouterde G, Barnetche T, et al. Short-term risk of total malignancy and nonmelanoma skin cancers with certolizumab and golimumab in patients with rheumatoid arthritis: metaanalysis of randomized controlled trials. J Rheumatol 2012;39:712–5.

41. Burmester GR, Panaccione R, Gordon KB, et al. Adalimumab: long-term safety in 23 458 patients from global clinical trials in rheumatoid arthritis, juvenile idiopathic arthritis, ankylosing spondylitis, psoriatic arthritis, psoriasis and Crohn's disease. Ann Rheum Dis 2013;72:517–24.

42. Mariette X, Reynolds AV, Emery P. Updated meta-analysis of non-melanoma skin cancer rates reported from prospective observational studies in patients treated with tumour necrosis factor inhibitors. Ann Rheum Dis 2012;71:e2.

43. Dreyer L, Mellemkjaer L, Andersen AR, et al. Incidences of overall and site specific cancers in TNFalpha inhibitor treated patients with rheumatoid arthritis and other arthritides - a follow-up study from the DANBIO Registry. Ann Rheum Dis 2013;72:79–82.

44. Raaschou P, Simard JF, Asker Hagelberg C, et al. Rheumatoid arthritis, anti-tumour necrosis factor treatment, and risk of squamous cell and basal cell skin cancer: cohort study based on nationwide prospectively recorded data from Sweden. BMJ 2016;352:i262.

45. Hoekstra HJ, Veerman K, van Ginkel RJ. Isolated limb perfusion for in-transit melanoma metastases: melphalan or TNF-melphalan perfusion? J Surg Oncol 2014; 109:338–47.

46. Deroose JP, Eggermont AM, van Geel AN, et al. Isolated limb perfusion for melanoma in-transit metastases: developments in recent years and the role of tumor necrosis factor alpha. Curr Opin Oncol 2011;23:183–8.

47. Raaschou P, Simard JF, Holmqvist M, et al. Rheumatoid arthritis, anti-tumour necrosis factor therapy, and risk of malignant melanoma: nationwide population based prospective cohort study from Sweden. BMJ 2013;346:f1939.
48. Mercer LK, Green AC, Galloway JB, et al. The influence of anti-TNF therapy upon incidence of keratinocyte skin cancer in patients with rheumatoid arthritis: longitudinal results from the British Society for Rheumatology Biologics Register. Ann Rheum Dis 2012;71(6):869–74.
49. Mercer LK, Askling J, Raaschou P, et al. Risk of invasive melanoma in patients with rheumatoid arthritis treated with biologics: results from a collaborative project of 11 European biologic registers. Ann Rheum Dis 2016. [Epub ahead of print].
50. Singh JA, Wells GA, Christensen R, et al. Adverse effects of biologics: a network meta-analysis and Cochrane overview. Cochrane Database Syst Rev 2011;(2):CD008794.
51. Weinblatt ME, Bathon JM, Kremer JM, et al. Safety and efficacy of etanercept beyond 10 years of therapy in North American patients with early and longstanding rheumatoid arthritis. Arthritis Care Res (Hoboken) 2011;63:373–82.
52. Kay J, Fleischmann R, Keystone E, et al. Golimumab 3-year safety update: an analysis of pooled data from the long-term extensions of randomised, double-blind, placebo-controlled trials conducted in patients with rheumatoid arthritis, psoriatic arthritis or ankylosing spondylitis. Ann Rheum Dis 2015;74:538–46.
53. Bykerk VP, Cush J, Winthrop K, et al. Update on the safety profile of certolizumab pegol in rheumatoid arthritis: an integrated analysis from clinical trials. Ann Rheum Dis 2015;74:96–103.
54. Smolen JS, Kay J, Doyle M, et al. Golimumab in patients with active rheumatoid arthritis after treatment with tumor necrosis factor alpha inhibitors: findings with up to five years of treatment in the multicenter, randomized, double-blind, placebo-controlled, phase 3 GO-AFTER study. Arthritis Res Ther 2015;17:14.
55. Mariette X, Tubach F, Bagheri H, et al. Lymphoma in patients treated with anti-TNF: results of the 3-year prospective French RATIO registry. Ann Rheum Dis 2010;69:400–8.
56. Morgan CL, Emery P, Porter D, et al. Treatment of rheumatoid arthritis with etanercept with reference to disease-modifying anti-rheumatic drugs: long-term safety and survival using prospective, observational data. Rheumatology (Oxford) 2014; 53:186–94.
57. Raaschou P, Frisell T, Askling J. TNF inhibitor therapy and risk of breast cancer recurrence in patients with rheumatoid arthritis: a nationwide cohort study. Ann Rheum Dis 2015;74:2137–43.
58. Strangfeld A, Hierse F, Rau R, et al. Risk of incident or recurrent malignancies among patients with rheumatoid arthritis exposed to biologic therapy in the German biologics register RABBIT. Arthritis Res Ther 2010;12:R5.
59. Dixon WG, Watson KD, Lunt M, et al. Influence of anti-tumor necrosis factor therapy on cancer incidence in patients with rheumatoid arthritis who have had a prior malignancy: results from the British Society for Rheumatology Biologics Register. Arthritis Care Res (Hoboken) 2010;62:755–63.
60. Strangfeld A, Pattloch D, Herzer P, et al. Risk of cancer recurrence or new tumors in RA patients with prior malignancies treated with various biologic agents. Arthritis Rheum 2013;65:806.
61. Poullenot F, Seksik P, Beaugerie L, et al. Risk of incident cancer in inflammatory bowel disease patients starting anti-TNF therapy while having recent malignancy. Inflamm Bowel Dis 2016;22(6):1362–9.

62. Mercer LK, Low AS, Galloway JB, et al. Anti-TNF therapy in women with rheumatoid arthritis with a history of carcinoma in situ of the cervix. Ann Rheum Dis 2013;72:143–4.

63. Cordtz R, Mellemkjaer L, Glintborg B, et al. Malignant progression of precancerous lesions of the uterine cervix following biological DMARD therapy in patients with arthritis. Ann Rheum Dis 2015;74:1479–80.

64. Wadstrom H, Frisell T, Sparen P, et al. Do RA or TNF inhibitors increase the risk of cervical neoplasia or of recurrence of previous neoplasia? A nationwide study from Sweden. Ann Rheum Dis 2016;75(7):1272–8.

65. Hooper M, Wenkert D, Bitman B, et al. Malignancies in children and young adults on etanercept: summary of cases from clinical trials and post marketing reports. Pediatr Rheumatol Online J 2013;11:35.

66. Diak P, Siegel J, La Gronade L, et al. Tumor necrosis factor alpha blockers and malignancy in children: forty-eight cases reported to the Food and Drug Administration. Arthritis Rheum 2010;62:2517–24.

67. Nordstrom BL, Mines D, Gu Y, et al. Risk of malignancy in children with juvenile idiopathic arthritis not treated with biologic agents. Arthritis Care Res (Hoboken) 2012;64:1357–64.

68. van Vollenhoven RF, Fleischmann RM, Furst DE, et al. Longterm safety of rituximab: final report of the Rheumatoid Arthritis Global Clinical Trial Program over 11 years. J Rheumatol 2015;42:1761–6.

69. Simon TA, Smitten AL, Franklin J, et al. Malignancies in the rheumatoid arthritis abatacept clinical development programme: an epidemiological assessment. Ann Rheum Dis 2009;68:1819–26.

70. Weinblatt ME, Moreland LW, Westhovens R, et al. Safety of abatacept administered intravenously in treatment of rheumatoid arthritis: integrated analyses of up to 8 years of treatment from the abatacept clinical trial program. J Rheumatol 2013;40:787–97.

71. Schiff MH, Kremer JM, Jahreis A, et al. Integrated safety in tocilizumab clinical trials. Arthritis Res Ther 2011;13:R141.

72. Rubbert-Roth A, Sebba A, Brockwell L, et al. Malignancy rates in patients with rheumatoid arthritis treated with tocilizumab. RMD Open 2016;2:e000213.

73. Yamamoto K, Goto H, Hirao K, et al. Longterm safety of tocilizumab: results from 3 years of followup postmarketing surveillance of 5573 patients with rheumatoid arthritis in Japan. J Rheumatol 2015;42:1368–75.

74. Yazici H, Yazici Y. Are we content that risk of cancer is not appreciably increased after tumor necrosis factor inhibitor use? Comment on the article by Solomon et al. Arthritis Rheum 2012;64:2414 [author reply: 5].

Immune-Related Adverse Effects of Cancer Immunotherapy— Implications for Rheumatology

Laura C. Cappelli, MD, MHS*, Ami A. Shah, MD, MHS,
Clifton O. Bingham III, MD

KEYWORDS

- Arthritis • Sicca syndrome • Immune checkpoint inhibitors • Malignancy
- Immune-related adverse events

KEY POINTS

- By blocking inhibitory pathways of T-cell activation, immune checkpoint inhibitors (ICIs) can cause immune-related adverse events (IRAEs), including inflammatory arthritis, myositis, vasculitis, and sicca syndrome.
- Treatment of ICI-induced rheumatic IRAE requires different considerations than treatment of classic rheumatic conditions.
- Using ICIs in those with preexisting autoimmunity is possible but with risk of causing a disease flare or a different IRAE.

INTRODUCTION

Interactions between the immune system and cancer are complex, dynamic, and bidirectional.[1] One of the primary roles of the immune system is to recognize and eliminate cells that have undergone malignant transformation, often before a developing tumor can become clinically apparent.[2] In some instances, successful tumor elimination does not occur, and a malignancy may be held in equilibrium where further tumor growth is prevented. Cancers that grow and reach clinical detection, however, have often developed successful strategies to evade naturally occurring host immune

Conflicts of Interest: Dr C.O. Bingham has served as a consultant for Bristol-Myers-Squibb.
Funding Sources: Dr L.C. Cappelli is supported by the Jerome L. Greene Foundation Scholar Award (# 90056963). Dr A.A. Shah is supported by National Institutes of Health, National Institute of Arthritis and Musculoskeletal and Skin Diseases (# K23-AR061439). Additional support was provided by a Jerome L. Greene Foundation Discovery Award and by RDRCC P30AR053503.
Division of Rheumatology, Johns Hopkins School of Medicine, 5501 Hopkins Bayview Circle, Suite 1.B1, Baltimore, MD, USA
* Corresponding author. Division of Rheumatology, Department of Medicine, Johns Hopkins University, 5200 Eastern Avenue, MFL Center Tower 4100, Baltimore, MD 21224.
E-mail address: lcappel1@jhmi.edu

responses. To combat this, immunotherapeutic agents are being used to harness the power of the immune system, by increasing the quality or quantity of immune effector cells, eliciting immune responses to specific tumor antigens, or inhibiting mechanisms that cancers develop to evade immunologic surveillance and killing mechanisms.[2]

Immunotherapy approaches to cancer began in the 1980s, when recombinant interleukin (IL)-2 was administered for metastatic melanoma with tumor regression seen in a subset of patients.[3] Since then, cancer vaccines and T-cell infusions have also been used successfully to treat a variety of malignancies. IL-2, T-cell infusions, and cancer vaccines all work by directly activating the immune system, thus augmenting host immune responses against malignancies. Another class of cancer therapies, the main focus of this article, works differently. These therapies, known as immune checkpoint inhibitors (ICI), work in part by targeting immunoregulatory pathways exploited by some cancers. Several inhibitory pathways, known as immunologic checkpoints, play critical roles in maintaining self-tolerance and preventing autoimmunity. Multiple tumor types, however, can appropriate immune checkpoint pathways to increase immune resistance in the tumor microenvironment.[4] T cells require both the interaction of the major histocompatibility complex molecule on an antigen-presenting cell (APC) with the T-cell receptor and the second signal of another ligand receptor interaction to become activated. An example of this is the interaction between B7 molecules (CD80/86) on APCs with CD28 on T cells. B7 can also bind instead to an inhibitory receptor, cytotoxic lymphocyte antigen 4 (CTLA-4) or CD154 (**Fig. 1A**). When this engagement occurs, the T cell does not become activated. Other immune checkpoints have also been identified and are targets for cancer immunotherapy. Another major immune checkpoint pathway is mediated through the programmed death protein-1 (PD-1) expressed on T cells and programmed death ligand (PD-L)1 expressed on APCs and also on many tumors, where it serves as to dampen the T-cell–mediated response and facilitate immunologic evasion[5] (see **Fig. 1A**). ICIs nonspecifically activate T cells by blocking negative costimulatory ligands or receptors on T cells, APCs, and/or tumor cells.[6]

Ipilimumab, a monoclonal antibody to CTLA-4, works by blocking the B7 binding to this down-regulatory receptor, thus leading to its unopposed engagement with the positive costimulatory receptor, CD28, and subsequent T-cell activation[7] (**Fig. 1B**). Agents, such as nivolomab and pembrolizumab; antibodies directed against PD-1; and atezolizumab, directed against PD-L1, block this additional inhibitory pathway leading to increased T-cell activation and can also interrupt down-regulatory signaling mediated through direct tumor–T-cell interactions (see **Fig. 1B**). The enhanced activation of T cells can enhance tumor targeting and killing but is not specific to only an antitumor response.

Currently, ICIs with 3 targets, CTLA-4, PD-1, and PD-L1, are Food and Drug Administration approved (**Table 1**). Ipilimumab, a CTLA-4 inhibitor, was the first approved for metastatic melanoma in 2011. Nivolumab, targeting PD-1, is approved for metastatic melanoma, non–small cell lung cancer (NSCLC), renal cell carcinoma (RCC), and Hodgkin lymphoma. Pembrolizumab, also a PD-1 inhibitor, is approved for metastatic melanoma and a subset of NSCLC. Atezolizumab, which blocks PD-L1, is approved for urothelial carcinoma. A combination regimen of ipilimumab and nivolumab is also approved for metastatic melanoma.

Currently approved ICIs provide a more effective therapeutic option for a variety of advanced stage cancers. In metastatic melanoma, ipilimumab, pembrolizumab, and nivolumab have shown significant survival benefits compared with traditional chemotherapy, with 5-year survival rates up to 25% to 31%.[7,8] In NSCLC, those treated

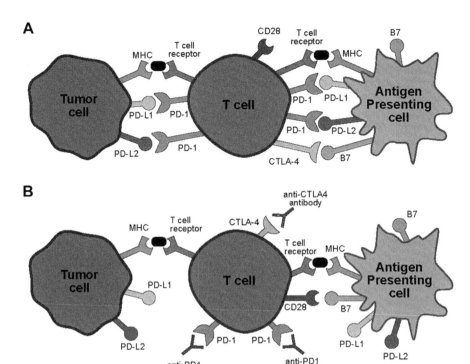

Fig. 1. Mechanism of action for immune checkpoint inhibition targeting CTLA-4 and PD-1. (*A*) Inhibition of T-cell activation by interactions with tumor cells and APCs. PD-L1 and PD-L2 on tumor cells and APCs bind to PD-1 on the T cell and B7 on APCs binds to CTLA-4 on the T cell. (*B*) Antibodies to PD-1 or CTLA-4 block inhibitory interactions, allowing for positive costimulation (B7 binds CD28).

with nivolumab had a 51% survival at 12 months compared with 39% with doce-taxel.[9] In RCC, there was nearly a 6-month survival benefit for nivolumab over chemotherapy.[10] Combination therapy targeting different checkpoints can be even more effective; treatment with ipilimumab and nivolumab for metastatic melanoma

Table 1
Approved immune checkpoint inhibitors and indications, targets of investigational drugs

Target	Food and Drug Administration–Approved Drugs	Drugs in Development (Partial List)
CTLA-4	Ipilimumab (Yervoy)—metastatic melanoma	Tremelimumab
PD-1	Nivolumab (Opdivo)—metastatic melanoma, NSCLC, renal cell carcinoma, Hodgkin lymphoma Pembrolizumab (Keytruda)—metastatic melanoma, PD-L1–positive NSCLC	Pidilizumab, AMP-224
PD-L1	Atezolizumab (Tecentriq) —urothelial carcinoma	Avelumab, Durvalumab
LAG-3	None	BMS-986016, IMP321
B7	None	Enoblituzumab, MGD009
TIM-3	None	MBG453
CD137	None	Urelumab

had a partial or total response rate of 60% in 1 study[11] compared with 11% with ipilimumab alone.

Due to these successes in melanoma, NSCLC, and RCC, there are many other ICI drugs currently in clinical trials, including drugs targeting PD-L1, T-cell immunoglobulin and mucin domain 3 (TIM-3), and lymphocyte activation gene 3 (LAG-3),[6] which represent other checkpoint pathways (see **Table 1**). In addition, these and currently approved ICIs are being studied in clinical trials alone and in combination, for a wide variety of cancers, from solid tumors to hematologic malignancies, and for cancer at various stages as part of initial regimens in addition to treatment of refractory disease.[6,12] With reports of efficacy in trials for diverse tumors like Merkel cell carcinoma[13] and a subset of colorectal cancer,[14] the approved indications of ICIs are likely to expand in the near future. With this expected increase in indications, many more people will be exposed to these therapies.

Why is this growth in the use of ICIs significant to the rheumatologist? ICIs can cause adverse effects through immune-mediated tissue damage known as IRAEs. These events vary widely in severity and can affect nearly any organ system. The incidence of IRAE varies by type of therapy and underlying malignancy.[15,16] Rash has been the most commonly reported event, in up to 30% to 35% of patients treated with PD-1 inhibitors for melanoma.[8] Cutaneous manifestations include vitiligo, neutrophilic dermatoses, pruritus, and toxic epidermal necrolysis.[17] Colitis and pneumonitis are less common, with incidence ranging from 1% to 5% in patients treated with anti–PD-1[9,10,18] or anti–CTLA-4[19,20] monotherapy. Both of these IRAEs can be severe, however, even resulting in death. Hepatitis, uveitis, pancreatitis, central nervous system disease, and peripheral neuropathies have also been reported.[21] Clinical manifestations of these IRAEs are described in **Table 2**. The time course for developing IRAEs is variable and can occur after 1 dose or after several months of therapy.[22] Skin manifestations and colitis tend to present early in therapy, whereas pneumonitis and endocrinopathies occur later.[22] As IRAEs are increasingly appreciated, musculoskeletal and rheumatic presentations are beginning to be described. These events, most likely to be seen by rheumatologists, are the focus of this article.

Table 2
Other (nonrheumatic or musculoskeletal) immune-related adverse events and clinical descriptions

Immune-related Adverse Events	Clinical Characteristics
Colitis	Diarrhea, in severe cases causing perforation or death. Usually develops earlier in therapy
Rash	Vitiligo, neutrophilic dermatoses, and other skin manifestations reported; develops early in therapy
Thyroiditis	Usually resulting in hypothyroidism; can be a late manifestation
Pneumonitis	Ranges from mild dyspnea and cough to hypoxic respiratory failure
Hypophysitis	Can affect all hormonal axes of anterior pituitary or can be selective; patients may need permanent hormone replacement
Hepatitis	Transaminitis, with or without elevated bilirubin
Central nervous system	Encephalopathy responsive to steroids has been reported
Peripheral nervous system	Peripheral neuropathy, Guillain-Barré syndrome reported

SPECTRUM AND INCIDENCE OF CURRENTLY DESCRIBED RHEUMATIC AND MUSCULOSKELETAL IMMUNE-RELATED ADVERSE EVENTS IN CLINICAL TRIALS

Arthralgia and arthritis are the most commonly reported rheumatic and musculo-skeletal IRAEs in ICI clinical trials to date. The incidence of arthralgia secondary to nivolumab in phase III trials ranges from 5% to 16%.[9] Similar rates have been reported with ipilimumab monotherapy.[23,24] Like other IRAEs, the incidence of arthralgia seems higher in combination ICI therapy, as was seen in a trial for melanoma where the ipilimumab group had a rate of arthralgia of 6.1%, the nivolumab group had an incidence of 7.7%, and the combination therapy group receiving ipilimumab and nivolumab was 10.5%.[23] When immunotherapy is combined with other modalities, like peptide vaccines, rates of arthralgia have been as reported as high as 43%.[25]

The incidence of true inflammatory arthritis is less clear. Arthritis is not always re-ported in publications of clinical trials, and there are several mutually exclusive ways to code musculoskeletal adverse events in the current systems used. For example, arthralgia, arthritis, joint effusion, and musculoskeletal pain are all potential options for coding an adverse event relating to the joint; thus, without any standardi-zation in place, the same symptom may be coded differently. This is illustrated in a phase I trial for nivolumab for advanced solid tumors, where 2 patients were reported as having "arthralgia," yet they were treated with corticosteroids, raising suspicion that these patients actually had inflammatory arthritis.[26]

Another issue that may contribute to lower reporting of musculoskeletal IRAE is the adverse event grading system used in oncologic trials. Many clinical trial reports only report adverse events of grade 3 or higher and do not mention events of lower severity. In the oncologic Common Terminology Criteria for Adverse Events (CTCAE), for arthritis, joint effusion, or arthralgia to reach a grade 3 for reporting requires hospital-ization for joint symptoms or for a patient to be nearly completely disabled. A working group within Outcome Measures in Rheumatology evaluated the oncologic CTCAE for its applicability in rheumatology settings.[27] In this exercise, adverse events coded in CTCAE were regraded, such that events causing impairment of function were up-coded to more severe ratings. Were such a schema in place, it is likely that the muscu-loskeletal and rheumatic adverse events in oncology trials would become more apparent and recognized in terms of their frequency and severity.

There are no observational studies of large cohorts that have systematically moni-tored patients for inflammatory arthritis with confirmation by rheumatologists. In 1 observational study, CT and PET/CT before and after therapy with CTLA-4 inhibitors were reviewed; 4 of 119 (3.4%) were reported as having arthritis on imaging.[28] Unfor-tunately, additional clinical information concerning the arthritis was limited. Further research is needed to identify how prevalent inflammatory arthritis is with different types of ICIs. The authors recently reported 9 cases of inflammatory arthritis second-ary to treatment of nivolumab and/or ipilimumab, but an appropriate denominator for incidence was difficult to calculate given the population of clinical trial participants and patients receiving therapy as standard of care, and not all cases occurring in patients in clinical trials could be reported due to publication embargoes.[29]

ICI-induced sicca syndrome has only been recently described as a clinical entity.[29] Dry mouth was reported in 24% of patients in a phase I trial of nivolumab and peptide vaccine for metastatic melanoma[25]; in a phase II trial of nivolumab for RCC, dose-related dry mouth occurred in 3% to 11% of patients.[30] In a trial of pembrolizumab versus ipilimumab in advanced melanoma, rates of dry mouth were 4% and 7% in the 2 dosing regimens of pembrolizumab.[18] Dry eyes were noted in 2 phase I trials of ipilimumab in combination with other therapies in 3%[31] and 4% of participants.[32] Neither the severity of symptoms nor treatment is apparent from the clinical trials.

Vasculitis has been rarely described in the ICI clinical trial literature. In a phase II trial of ipilimumab with and without dacarbazine for melanoma, 1 case of grade 2 autoimmune vasculitis was reported among 74 patients treated, but no further clinical description is provided.[33] In a phase I trial of ipilimumab with and without bevacizumab for metastatic melanoma, 1 case of giant cell arteritis developed among 46 patients treated.[32]

Myalgia and muscle weakness have been reported as adverse events in clinical trials. Myalgia was seen in 2% to 18% of participants in trials of nivolumab[25,34] and ipilimumab,[32] whereas muscle weakness was reported in 1% of patients in a phase II trial of ipilimumab with and without sargramostim[30] and 12% of patients in a phase I trial of nivolumab and peptide vaccine.[25] The clinical descriptions of these events cannot be discerned from the clinical trials to determine if these could have potentially been related to inflammatory muscle disease. Cases of inflammatory myositis have been subsequently reported and are discussed in more detail later.

A single case of lupus nephritis after treatment with ipilimumab has been reported, but no cases of ICI-induced systemic lupus erythematous affecting other organ systems have been noted. Scleroderma secondary to ICIs has also not been reported.

CLINICAL FEATURES OF RHEUMATIC IMMUNE-RELATED ADVERSE EVENTS
Inflammatory Arthritis

Two cases of inflammatory arthritis and tenosynovitis after pembrolizumab therapy have been reported.[35] Both patients were seronegative (for rheumatoid factor [RF] and anticyclic citrullinated peptide [CCP] antibodies) and had involvement of large joints. One patient also had involvement of the proximal interphalageal joints. MRI of these 2 patients showed synovitis in the ankle and wrist with enhancement in the tendons consistent with tenosynovitis. For 1 patient pembrolizumab was held and nonsteroidal anti-inflammatory drugs (NSAIDs) used with improvement of the arthritis; the other was managed with pembrolizumab cessation and NSAIDs and hydroxychloroquine.

A case of Jaccoud arthropathy and uveitis after treatment with nivolumab for RCC has been described.[36] The patient initially developed uveitis, which responded to intraocular steroids. This was followed by morning stiffness and reducible swan neck deformities in the hands. No erosions were seen on radiographs of the hands, and antinuclear antibody (ANA) was negative. Treatment of the arthropathy was not described.

The authors have recently reported 3 subtypes of inflammatory arthritis[29] in 9 patients treated with ipilimumab, nivolumab, or combination therapy. These subtypes are a polyarthritis similar to rheumatoid arthritis, true reactive arthritis with conjunctivitis, urethritis and oligoarthritis, and a subtype similar to seronegative spondyloarthritis with inflammatory back pain and predominantly larger joint involvement. The arthritis was often additive; patients would start with 1 or 2 affected joints and progress to a highly inflammatory polyarthritis. Although most patients have been seronegative, 1 patient had a positive RF, and 3 patients had positive ANAs, most of low titer. MRI and ultrasound confirmed synovitis in several patients. Four patients had synovial fluid analysis, all of which was inflammatory with 9000 cells/mL to 30,000 white blood cells/mL and a neutrophilic predominance. In contrast to the patients previously described who experienced polyarthritis from pembrolizumab that responded to NSAIDs and hydroxychloroquine, 8 of 9 of this group of patients required systemic corticosteroids for improvement in their symptoms. Doses of steroids were as high as 120 mg daily. Three patients required tumor necrosis factor (TNF) inhibitors to control their symptoms.

Sicca Syndrome

The only report of sicca syndrome secondary to ICIs to date is 4 cases of severe salivary hypofunction after treatment with nivolumab, ipilimumab, or combination therapy.[29] The dry mouth symptoms were more severe than dry eyes in all 4 patients. All patients were negative for Ro antibodies, whereas 1 patient was positive for La/SS-B antibodies and had parotitis with a parotid ultrasound showing hypoechoic foci. The patient with parotitis was treated with 6 weeks of prednisone, tapering from 40 mg daily, that resulted in resolution of parotid swelling.

Myositis

Two cases of inflammatory myopathy from ICIs have been reported. One case was more consistent with dermatomyositis,[37] where the patient had proximal muscle weakness, a heliotrope rash and V-neck sign (erythematous rash of the chest), and an elevated creatinine kinase (CK) level of 1854 U/L. She was treated with prednisone, 80 mg daily, with normalization of her CK. The prednisone was tapered off after 8 weeks and ipilimumab was discontinued. The other case occurred after nivolumab therapy for metastatic melanoma.[38] This patient had respiratory muscle involvement along with proximal muscle weakness and an elevated CK of 2812 U/L. Nivolumab was stopped, and he received 5 days of prednisone, 30 mg daily, with eventual improvement. There is also a case of eosinophilic fasciitis, which can be a myositis mimic, secondary to pembrolizumab.[39]

Vasculitis

Two cases of giant cell arteritis/polymyalgia rheumatica after ipilimumab for metastatic melanoma have been described.[40] Both patients had temporal artery biopsies confirming the diagnosis and responded to treatment with prednisone, 50 mg to 60 mg daily. Single-organ vasculitis from ICIs is also possible because retinal[41] vasculitis and uterine[42] vasculitis have been seen after pembrolizumab and ipilimumab, respectively.

Lupus Nephritis

One case of lupus nephritis associated with ICI treatment has been reported in a patient treated with ipilimumab for metastatic melanoma.[43] When new nephrotic range proteinuria developed, a kidney biopsy was performed with immunofluorescence positive for IgM, IgG, C3, and C1q in the mesangial space. Antibodies to double-stranded DNA were positive initially and negative when checked after discontinuation of ipilimumab. Proteinuria persisted, however, and a venous thrombosis of the left kidney was discovered. After anticoagulation and prednisone therapy, the patient improved.

EVALUATION OF SUSPECTED RHEUMATIC IMMUNE-RELATED ADVERSE EVENTS

For patients with suspected rheumatic IRAE, the authors recommend a full evaluation with a rheumatologist focusing on clinical characteristics, laboratory testing, imaging, and other specific tests as outlined in **Table 3**. Because the phenotypes of rheumatic IRAE are not fully understood, learning about which ways IRAE are similar to or different from autoimmune diseases not related to ICIs can potentially be helpful in

Table 3
Recommendations for evaluation of patients with suspected rheumatic immune-related adverse events

Suspected Immune-related Adverse Event	Clinical Examination	Laboratory Studies	Imaging, Other Studies
Inflammatory arthritis	Full joint examination Schober test	ESR, CRP, RF, CCP, ANA, HLA B27	Synovial fluid analysis Joint ultrasound or MRI
Sicca syndrome	Schirmer test Palpation of parotid glands Unstimulated salivary flow assessment	ESR, CRP, ANA, Ro, La	Parotid gland ultrasound Salivary scintigram Minor salivary gland biopsy
Myositis	Manual strength testing Dynamometry	CK, aldolase, ESR, CRP, ANA Myositis panel (Jo-1, PL-7, PL-12, EJ, OJ, Mi-2, SRP)	Electromyography MRI of affected muscle
Vasculitis	GCA: palpation of temporal arteries Palpation and auscultation of arteries Skin examination (purpura) Evaluation for mononeuritis multiplex	ESR, CRP, cANCA, pANCA, MPO, PR3, urinalysis	For GCA: temporal artery biopsy MRI or PET of suspected affected area

Abbreviations: ANA, anti-nuclear antibodies; cANCA, cytoplasmic anti-neutrophil cytoplasmic antibodies; CCP, cyclic citrullinated peptide antibodies; CRP, C-reactive protein; ESR, erythrocyte sedimentation rate; GCA, giant cell arteritis; HLA, human leukocyte antigen; pANCA, perinuclear anti-neutrophil cytoplasmic antibodies; PR3, proteinase-3; RF, rheumatoid factor; MPO, myeloperoxidase.

guiding treatment. Because autoantibody formation is a possible mechanism for the development of IRAE, as shown in hypophysitis,[44] relevant autoantibodies should be evaluated for suspected inflammatory arthritis, sicca syndrome, vasculitis, or myositis (see **Table 3**). The authors recommend evaluating for autoantibodies, although in the authors' experience to date and in the cases reported, traditional serologic markers may be negative. The lack of traditional autoantibodies may suggest a unique mechanism for rheumatic IRAE. Also, the highly inflammatory nature of the syndromes seems to be distinct raising the question of nonspecific activation of both immunologic and inflammatory cascades.

TREATMENT CONSIDERATIONS

No treatment algorithms currently exist for treatment of rheumatic and musculoskeletal IRAEs. For other IRAEs, like colitis, pneumonitis, dermatologic manifestations, and hepatitis, treatment recommendations have been developed based on clinical experience.[15,45] These treatment algorithms give recommendations based on the grade of adverse event about treating with corticosteroids, TNF inhibitors, and holding or stopping the ICI.

Extrapolating from these algorithms, the authors suggest basing treatment on symptom severity and functional consequences (**Fig. 2**). NSAIDs and low-dose corticosteroids can be used for patients with milder symptoms, with intra-articular corticosteroids also an option for significantly symptomatic joints. Increased dose of corticosteroids, up to 1 mg/kg to 1.5 mg/kg daily of prednisone, may be needed for severe cases. In those who are refractory to prednisone or who cannot be tapered, starting TNF inhibitors is the next recommendation. Based on the responses seen with TNF inhibitors for ICI-related colitis and the authors' own experience, TNF inhibitors seem a reasonable next step in those who have failed steroid tapers. There are some hypothetical concerns about long-term effects of these medications on cancer progression given their association with nonmelanoma skin cancer and possible association with melanoma in rheumatoid arthritis[46] and the association with solid tumors seen in a trial of etanercept for granulomatosis with polyangiitis.[47] Infliximab has been used over short periods of time to treat ICI-induced colitis in metastatic melanoma with no ill effects[48] but has not been used in extended courses. The authors do not recommend using abatacept because it directly opposes the mechanism of ICIs. Given the colitis that is possible with ICIs, there are considerable concerns about using tocilizumab and tofacitinib given the concerns of colonic perforation with IL-6 and JAK inhibition. The introduction of biologic agents requires careful evaluation of benefits versus potential risks in consultation with the patient's treating oncologist.

Hydroxychloroquine, sulfasalazine, methotrexate, and other nonbiologic disease-modifying antirheumatic drugs can be considered because they are less likely to raise

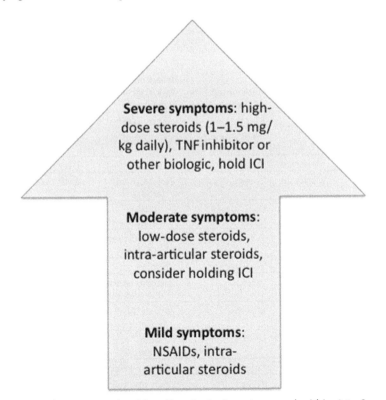

Severe symptoms: high-dose steroids (1–1.5 mg/kg daily), TNF inhibitor or other biologic, hold ICI

Moderate symptoms: low-dose steroids, intra-articular steroids, consider holding ICI

Mild symptoms: NSAIDs, intra-articular steroids

Fig. 2. Proposed treatment algorithm. If patients do not respond within 4 to 6 weeks of therapy, escalate to next level of treatment.

tumor risk or interfere with therapy (**Table 4**). One consideration with these therapies, however, is their slow onset of action (given the fulminant articular presentations seen thus far). In patients with a potentially limited life expectancy, they may fail to achieve optimal effect quickly enough to improve the impairments in quality of life. Similarly, any treatment that is started in patients with rheumatic IRAE should be re-evaluated for response, in approximately 4 to 6 weeks, and switched to a different modality if there is not improvement.

OTHER CONSIDERATIONS

- Metastatic disease: for patients with inflammatory arthritis, if a single joint is disproportionately affected or not improving with therapy, imaging to evaluate for bony metastasis should be performed. This has been reported in a patient with elbow arthritis.[29]
- Treatment length: there is uncertainty about how long to continue treatment in patients with rheumatic IRAE. In other nonrheumatic IRAE, some are self-limited or respond quickly to treatment whereas others can be persistent.[22]
- Relationship between IRAE and tumor response: the relationship between development of an IRAE secondary to ICI therapy has not been definitively linked to improved tumor regression. It has been appreciated, however, that those treated

Table 4
Potential immunosuppressive therapy for immune checkpoint inhibitors–induced rheumatic immune-related adverse events

Drug Options	Likelihood of Efficacy	Anticipated Time of Onset	Effect on Cancer Risk/Cancer Response	Potential Side Effects (Overlap with Immune Checkpoint Inhibitors)
HCQ	Low	Months	Likely no effect	None
Sulfasalazine	Low	Weeks–months	Likely no effect	Allergic reaction/rash?
Methotrexate	Moderate	Weeks–months	Likely no effect	Liver toxicity
Leflunomide	Moderate	Weeks–months	Possible T-cell target	Liver toxicity
TNF inhibitors	High	Days–weeks	Possible melanoma risk	None
Abatacept	High	Weeks	*Likely impaired response*	None
Tocilizumab	High	Weeks	Unclear	*GI issues, colitis*
Tofacitinib (JAK inhibitors)	High	Weeks	Possible natural killer–cell target	*GI issues, colitis*
Azathioprine	Moderate	Months	Possible T-cell target	GI issues?
Mycophenolate	Moderate	Weeks–months	Possible T-cell target	GI issues?
Anakinra	Moderate	Days	Likely no effect	None
Secukinumab	Moderate	Weeks	Likely no effect	None

Drugs to avoid are listed in italic.
Abbreviation: GI, gastrointestinal.

with interferon for melanoma who exhibit signs of autoimmunity have an improvement in survival,[49] so this association is theoretically possible.

- Quality of life: patients have been very disabled as a result of rheumatic and musculoskeletal IRAE. Having discussions with patients about their goals and wishes is paramount, especially given that many have a limited life span.

IMMUNE CHECKPOINT INHIBITION IN PATIENTS WITH KNOWN AUTOIMMUNE DISEASE

The initial trials of ICIs excluded patients with preexisting autoimmune disease, so there are few data on how these drugs affect this group of patients. Now that several therapies are approved, case reports and 1 observational study of patients can provide some guidance on how to manage patients with preexisting autoimmune disease. For inflammatory bowel disease (IBD), pretreatment endoscopy to confirm that the IBD was not active allowed for successful use of ipilimumab for metastatic melanoma in 1 case report.[50] Another patient with ulcerative colitis was treated with ipilimumab for metastatic melanoma and developed severe colitis requiring colectomy.[51]

An observational study of 30 patients with various autoimmune diseases (rheumatoid arthritis, psoriasis, IBD, systemic lupus erythematosus, multiple sclerosis, autoimmune thyroid disease, sarcoidosis, and others) who received ipilimumab as standard of care was published in 2015.[52] Of the 30 patients, 8 had a flare of their underlying autoimmune disease that could be managed with corticosteroids. Ten patients had a conventional IRAE, like colitis or hyophysitis, and 1 patient died of presumptive ICI-induced colitis. Fifteen of the 30 did not have an IRAE or flare of their underlying disease. Six of the patients had a complete or partial response of their malignancy to therapy. From these data, it seems that it is possible to treat patients with a history of autoimmune disease with ICIs but with careful monitoring because the rate of flare and conventional IRAEs is substantial.

FUTURE DIRECTIONS FOR CLINICAL PRACTICE AND RESEARCH

There are several features of rheumatic IRAEs that merit further study. Pathogenesis of rheumatic IRAE is unclear and will likely differ from classical autoimmune diseases. The optimal timing of treatment (eg, induction, tapering) is unknown as are the true clinical spectrum of illness and risk factors for developing IRAE. Concerns with immunosuppressive agents increasing risk of tumor recurrence must also be evaluated. Addressing these issues will require a concerted effort involving rheumatology and oncology investigators, well-characterized patient phenotypes, and examination of potential mechanisms for the development of these events. Understanding risk factors for developing an IRAE can help risk stratify individuals at the start of therapy and influence clinical monitoring. Optimal treatment will require in-depth discussions between rheumatology and oncology concerning the risks vs benefits and likelihood of success for treatment of the underlying malignancy and with patients concerning overall quality of life. The advances in immunologic understanding related to the bidirectional relationships between autoimmunity and cancer[53,54] provide an important basis for investigation and should help to further understanding of the immunologic continuum to develop optimal strategies.

SUMMARY

ICIs will be increasingly used as they are approved for more tumor types and for use in combination, and as novel therapies targeting other immune checkpoint molecules are also approved. As use increases, there is a great likelihood that patients will be referred to rheumatology for evaluation and longitudinal management. Recognizing these syndromes and rapidly initiating therapy may help improve quality of life for affected patients. With careful evaluation of larger cohorts of patients, the incidence of rheumatic and musculoskeletal IRAE will be better defined and the mechanisms may be better understood.

REFERENCES

1. Shah AA, Casciola-Rosen L, Rosen A. Review: cancer-induced autoimmunity in the rheumatic diseases. Arthritis Rheumatol 2015;67(2):317–26.
2. Schreiber RD, Old LJ, Smyth MJ. Cancer immunoediting: integrating immunity's roles in cancer suppression and promotion. Science 2011;331(6024):1565–70.
3. Rosenberg SA. IL-2: the first effective immunotherapy for human cancer. J Immunol 2014;192(12):5451–8.
4. Pardoll DM. The blockade of immune checkpoints in cancer immunotherapy. Nat Rev Cancer 2012;12(4):252–64.
5. Brahmer JR, Hammers H, Lipson EJ. Nivolumab: targeting PD-1 to bolster anti-tumor immunity. Future Oncol 2015;11(9):1307–26.
6. Topalian SI, Drake CG, Pardoll DM. Immune checkpoint blockade: a common denominator approach to cancer therapy. Cancer Cell 2015;27(4):450–61.
7. Buchbinder EI, McDermott DF. Cytotoxic T-lymphocyte antigen-4 blockade in melanoma. Clin Ther 2015;37(4):755–63.
8. Ivashko IN, Kolesar JM. Pembrolizumab and nivolumab: PD-1 inhibitors for advanced melanoma. Am J Health Syst Pharm 2016;73(4):193–201.
9. Brahmer J, Reckamp KL, Baas P, et al. Nivolumab versus docetaxel in advanced squamous-cell non-small-cell lung cancer. N Engl J Med 2015;373(2):123–35.
10. Motzer RJ, Escudier B, McDermott DF, et al. Nivolumab versus everolimus in advanced renal-cell carcinoma. N Engl J Med 2015;373(19):1803–13.
11. Postow MA, Chesney J, Pavlick AC, et al. Nivolumab and ipilimumab versus ipilimumab in untreated melanoma. N Engl J Med 2015;372(21):2006–17.
12. NIH. ClinialTrials.gov website. 2015. Available at: https://clinicaltrials.gov/. Accessed December 27, 2015.
13. Nghiem PT, Bhatia S, Lipson EJ, et al. PD-1 Blockade with pembrolizumab in advanced Merkel-cell carcinoma. N Engl J Med 2016;374:2542–52.
14. Le DT, Uram JN, Wang H, et al. PD-1 Blockade in tumors with mismatch-repair deficiency. N Engl J Med 2015;372(26):2509–20.
15. Weber JS, Yang JC, Atkins MB, et al. Toxicities of immunotherapy for the practitioner. J Clin Oncol 2015;33(18):2092–9.
16. Naidoo J, Page DB, Li BT, et al. Toxicities of the anti-PD-1 and anti-PD-L1 immune checkpoint antibodies. Ann Oncol 2015;26(12):2375–91.
17. Spain L, Diem S, Larkin J. Management of toxicities of immune checkpoint inhibitors. Cancer Treat Rev 2016;44:51–60.
18. Robert C, Schachter J, Long GV, et al. Pembrolizumab versus ipilimumab in advanced melanoma. N Engl J Med 2015;372(26):2521–32.
19. Wolchok JD, Neyns B, Linette G, et al. Ipilimumab monotherapy in patients with pretreated advanced melanoma: a randomised, double-blind, multicentre, phase 2, dose-ranging study. Lancet Oncol 2010;11(2):155–64.
20. Hodi FS, O'Day SJ, McDermott DF, et al. Improved survival with ipilimumab in patients with metastatic melanoma. N Engl J Med 2010;363(8):711–23.
21. Postow MA. Managing immune checkpoint-blocking antibody side effects. Am Soc Clin Oncol Educ Book 2015;35:76–83.

22. Weber JS, Kahler KC, Hauschild A. Management of immune-related adverse events and kinetics of response with ipilimumab. J Clin Oncol 2012;30(21): 2691–7.

23. Larkin J, Chiarion-Sileni V, Gonzalez R, et al. Combined nivolumab and ipilimumab or monotherapy in untreated melanoma. N Engl J Med 2015;373(1):23–34.

24. Kwon ED, Drake CG, Scher HI, et al. Ipilimumab versus placebo after radiotherapy in patients with metastatic castration-resistant prostate cancer that had progressed after docetaxel chemotherapy (CA184-043): a multicentre, randomised, double-blind, phase 3 trial. Lancet Oncol 2014;15(7):700–12.

25. Gibney GT, Kudchadkar RR, DeConti RC, et al. Safety, correlative markers, and clinical results of adjuvant nivolumab in combination with vaccine in resected high-risk metastatic melanoma. Clin Cancer Res 2015;21(4):712–20.

26. Brahmer JR, Drake CG, Wollner I, et al. Phase I study of single-agent anti-programmed death-1 (MDX-1106) in refractory solid tumors: safety, clinical activity, pharmacodynamics, and immunologic correlates. J Clin Oncol 2010;28(19): 3167–75.

27. Woodworth T, Furst DE, Alten R, et al. Standardizing assessment and reporting of adverse effects in rheumatology clinical trials II: the rheumatology common toxicity criteria v.2.0. J Rheumatol 2007;34(6):1401–14.

28. Bronstein Y, Ng CS, Hwu P, et al. Radiologic manifestations of immune-related adverse events in patients with metastatic melanoma undergoing anti-CTLA-4 antibody therapy. AJR Am J Roentgenol 2011;197(6):W992–1000.

29. Capozzi V, Makhoul S, Aprea E, et al. PTR-MS characterization of VOCs associated with commercial aromatic bakery yeasts of wine and beer origin. Molecules 2016;21(4):483.

30. Motzer RJ, Rini BI, McDermott DF, et al. Nivolumab for metastatic renal cell carcinoma: results of a randomized phase II trial. J Clin Oncol 2015;33(13):1430–7.

31. Le DT, Lutz E, Uram JN, et al. Evaluation of ipilimumab in combination with allogeneic pancreatic tumor cells transfected with a GM-CSF gene in previously treated pancreatic cancer. J Immunother 2013;36(7):382–9.

32. Hodi FS, Lee S, McDermott DF, et al. Ipilimumab plus sargramostim vs ipilimumab alone for treatment of metastatic melanoma: a randomized clinical trial. JAMA 2014;312(17):1744–53.

33. Hersh EM, O'Day SJ, Powderly J, et al. A phase II multicenter study of ipilimumab with or without dacarbazine in chemotherapy-naive patients with advanced melanoma. Invest New Drugs 2011;29(3):489–98.

34. Borghaei H, Paz-Ares L, Horn L, et al. Nivolumab versus docetaxel in advanced nonsquamous non-small-cell lung cancer. N Engl J Med 2015;373(17):1627–39.

35. Chan MM, Kefford RF, Carlino M, et al. Arthritis and tenosynovitis associated with the anti-PD1 antibody pembrolizumab in metastatic melanoma. J Immunother 2015;38(1):37–9.

36. de Velasco G, Bermas B, Choueiri TK. Auto-immune arthropathy and uveitis as complications from PD-1 inhibitor. Arthritis Rheumatol 2016;68:556–7.

37. Sheik Ali S, Goddard AL, Luke JJ, et al. Drug-associated dermatomyositis following ipilimumab therapy: a novel immune-mediated adverse event associated with cytotoxic T-lymphocyte antigen 4 blockade. JAMA Dermatol 2015; 151(2):195–9.

38. Yoshioka M, Kambe N, Yamamoto Y, et al. Case of respiratory discomfort due to myositis after administration of nivolumab. J Dermatol 2015;42(10):1008–9.

39. Khoja L, Maurice C, Chappell M, et al. Eosinophilic fasciitis and acute encephalopathy toxicity from pembrolizumab treatment of a patient with metastatic melanoma. Cancer Immunol Res 2016;4:175–8.

40. Goldstein BL, Gedmintas L, Todd DJ. Drug-associated polymyalgia rheumatica/giant cell arteritis occurring in two patients after treatment with ipilimumab, an antagonist of ctla-4. Arthritis Rheumatol 2014;66(3):768–9.

41. Manusow JS, Khoja L, Pesin N, et al. Retinal vasculitis and ocular vitreous metastasis following complete response to PD-1 inhibition in a patient with metastatic cutaneous melanoma. J Immunother Cancer 2014;2(1):41.

42. Minor DR, Bunker SR, Doyle J. Lymphocytic vasculitis of the uterus in a patient with melanoma receiving ipilimumab. J Clin Oncol 2013;31(20):e356.

43. Fadel F, El Karoui K, Knebelmann B. Anti-CTLA4 antibody-induced lupus nephritis. N Engl J Med 2009;361(2):211–2.

44. Iwama S, De Remigis A, Callahan MK, et al. Pituitary expression of CTLA-4 mediates hypophysitis secondary to administration of CTLA-4 blocking antibody. Sci Transl Med 2014;6(230):230ra245.

45. Klair JS, Girotra M, Hutchins LF, et al. Ipilimumab-induced gastrointestinal toxicities: a management algorithm. Dig Dis Sci 2016;61:2132–9.

46. Turesson C, Matteson EL. Malignancy as a comorbidity in rheumatic diseases. Rheumatology (Oxford) 2013;52(1):5–14.

47. Stone JH, Holbrook JT, Marriott MA, et al. Solid malignancies among patients in the Wegener's Granulomatosis Etanercept Trial. Arthritis Rheum 2006;54(5):1608–18.

48. Johnston RL, Lutzky J, Chodhry A, et al. Cytotoxic T-lymphocyte-associated antigen 4 antibody-induced colitis and its management with infliximab. Dig Dis Sci 2009;54(11):2538–40.

49. Gogas H, Ioannovich J, Dafni U, et al. Prognostic significance of autoimmunity during treatment of melanoma with interferon. N Engl J Med 2006;354(7):709–18.

50. Gielisse EA, de Boer NK. Ipilimumab in a patient with known Crohn's disease: to give or not to give? J Crohns Colitis 2014;8(12):1742.

51. Bostwick AD, Salama AK, Hanks BA. Rapid complete response of metastatic melanoma in a patient undergoing ipilimumab immunotherapy in the setting of active ulcerative colitis. J Immunother Cancer 2015;3:19.

52. Johnson DB, Sullivan RJ, Ott PA, et al. Ipilimumab therapy in patients with advanced melanoma and preexisting autoimmune disorders. JAMA Oncol 2016;2:234–40.

53. Joseph CG, Darrah E, Shah AA, et al. Association of the autoimmune disease scleroderma with an immunologic response to cancer. Science 2014;343(6167):152–7.

54. Shah AA, Rosen A, Hummers L, et al. Close temporal relationship between onset of cancer and scleroderma in patients with RNA polymerase I/III antibodies. Arthritis Rheum 2010;62(9):2787–95.

Malignancy and Janus Kinase Inhibition

Padmapriya Sivaraman, MD[a,b,c,*], Stanley B. Cohen, MD[a,b,c]

KEYWORDS

- Malignancy • Rheumatoid arthritis • Jak inhibitors • Tofacitinib • Lymphoma
- Lung cancer

KEY POINTS

- Janus kinase inhibitors have been shown to be effective for treatment of rheumatoid arthritis (RA).
- The risk of malignancy in patients with RA treated with tofacitinib is similar to what has been reported with disease-modifying antirheumatic drugs and biologics.
- The risk of malignancy with tofacitinib in the RA population was not dose related except for an increased risk of nonmelanoma skin cancers in the long-term extension studies with the 10-mg dose.
- Based on clinical trial and long-term extension data, the rate of malignancy in patients with RA treated with tofacitinib does not increase over time with treatment.
- Based on clinical trial and long-term extension data, the risk of malignancy with tofacitinib treatment is similar to what is expected in the RA population.

INTRODUCTION

The management of rheumatoid arthritis (RA) has dramatically transformed over the last 20 years. The use of early aggressive therapy targeting low disease activity and the development of biologic therapies has dramatically improved patient outcomes with slowing of structural damage, improved physical function, and prolonged survival.[1–4]

However, biologic therapies have limitations; more than half of the patients continue to have active disease and require either subcutaneous or intravenous administration; they are associated with significant expense; and they can induce immunogenicity. Over the last 25 years, the intracellular signaling pathways involved in signal transduction from the cell surface to the nucleus after ligand-receptor binding have been

[a] Department of Internal Medicine, University of Texas Southwestern Medical School, 5323 Harry Hines Blvd, Dallas, TX 75390, USA; [b] Division of Rheumatology, Presbyterian Hospital, 8200 Walnut Hill Ln, Dallas, TX 75231, USA; [c] Metroplex Clinical Research Center, 8144 Walnut Hill Ln, #800, Dallas, TX 75231, USA
* Corresponding author. Department of Internal Medicine, University of Texas Southwestern Medical School, Dallas, TX.
E-mail address: psivaraman@arthdocs.com

Rheum Dis Clin N Am 43 (2017) 79–93
http://dx.doi.org/10.1016/j.rdc.2016.09.008
0889-857X/17/© 2016 Elsevier Inc. All rights reserved.

identified. This improved understanding of these pathways has provided opportunities for development of small molecule therapies that could target these pathways modifying proinflammatory cytokine production. Multiple preclinical studies have shown benefit in inhibiting various intracellular kinases, such as p38 Map kinase, and SyK (spleen tyrosine kinases) but failed to show benefit in RA clinical trials.[5]

In 2012, tofacitinib, an oral Janus kinase (Jak) inhibitor, was approved for RA treatment and other Jak inhibitors are under development, with baricitinib recently completing phase III trials in RA and selective inhibitors for Jak1 in phase II/III trials.[6] Jaks are protein tyrosine kinases that bind the cytoplasmic region of transmembrane cytokine receptors and mediate signaling through type I and type II cytokine receptors. After receptor-ligand interaction, various Jaks are activated, resulting in tyrosine phosphorylation of the receptor and subsequent activation of STATs (signal transducer and activators of transcription), which act as transcription factors. Jak/STAT signaling mediates cellular responses to multiple cytokines and growth factors. These responses include proliferation, differentiation, migration, apoptosis, and cell survival, depending on the signal and cellular context. Activated STATs enter the nucleus and bind to specific enhancer sequences in target genes, affecting their transcription.[7] Jaks consists of 4 types: Jak1, Jak2, Jak3, and Tyk2. The JAKs signal as pairs. Jak3 is primarily expressed in hematopoietic cells and is critical for signal transduction from the common gamma chain of the receptors for interleukin (IL)-2, IL-4, IL-7, IL-9, IL-15, and IL-21 on the plasma membrane to the nuclei of immune cells. Jak3 only signals in combination with Jak1. The cytokines are integral to lymphocyte activation, function, and proliferation. Jak3-knockout mice have defects in T and B lymphocytes and natural killer cells, with no other defects reported. Humans lacking Jak3 develop a severe combined immunodeficiency with a deficiency in natural killer cells and T lymphocytes.[8] Tofacitinib is a more selective inhibitor of Jak3/Jak1 based on enzymatic/cellular assays, but at the serum levels that have been achieved it also has an impact on Jak2.[9]

Jak1 and Jak2 were initially not considered as potential therapeutic targets because knocking out these kinases results in germline lethality. Baricitinib, which is a Jak1/Jak2 inhibitor, is in development for RA and has shown similar efficacy and safety to tofacitinib. Ruxolitinib, which has selectivity for Jak1/Jak2 is approved for myelofibrosis.[10,11] Hormones like the cytokines erythropoietin, thrombopoietin, growth hormone, granulocyte-macrophage colony-stimulating factor, IL-3, and IL-5 all signal through Jak2. IL-6, IL-10, IL-11, IL-19, IL-20, IL-22, and interferons gamma, alfa, and beta signal through Jak1. Tyk2 facilitates signaling for IL-12, IL-23, and type 1 interferons.[12] Tyk2 pairs with either Jak1 or Jak2 to facilitate signaling. At present, no specific Tyk2 inhibitors are under development for RA.[13,14]

Tofacitinib was approved by the US Food and Drug Administration (FDA) for patients with RA with active disease despite methotrexate treatment at a dosage of 5 mg twice daily in combination with nonbiologic disease-modifying antirheumatic drugs (DMARDs) or as monotherapy. The American College of Rheumatology guidelines recommend the use for moderate to severe RA that is nonresponsive to conventional DMARDs, and additionally also recommended their continued long-term use in patients who attain clinical remission.[15]

RA and other autoimmune conditions are chronic inflammatory states and are characterized by abnormalities of the immune system. Treatment of RA consists of medications that alter the upregulated immune system. The immune system is thought to play an important role in immune surveillance and protection from development of malignancy, with increased risk of certain malignancies, such as lymphomas, lung cancer, and nonmelanoma skin cancers (NMSCs), in patients with RA compared with the general population.[16] The available information on Jak inhibition and the potential development of malignancies are reviewed here and the risk of malignancies is compared with that reported with biologic therapies.

OVERALL MALIGNANCY RISK IN RHEUMATOID ARTHRITIS

As a background to understanding the risk of malignancy and Jak inhibition it is important to examine what is known about malignancy risk in RA and there are still gaps in the knowledge on this issue. It remains unclear whether the perceived risk for malignancies in RA is related to the underlying chronic inflammatory state, immunologic stimulation (suppression of T cells and malignant transformation of CD5 B cells), the use of biologics/nonbiologic DMARDs, or a result of a combination of the these factors.[16–18] The overall risk of malignancy in adult patients with RA is thought to be similar to that of the general population, based on observational databases.[16,19–21] Data using the general population as a comparator group in various RA studies in the United States were obtained from the Surveillance, Epidemiology and End Results (SEER) program of the National Cancer Institute database.[22] In general, the overall pooled standardized incidence ratio (SIR) for malignancies in RA is 1.09 (95% confidence interval [CI], 1.06–1.13) compared with the general population.[19] However, patients with RA seem to have a higher risk for certain site-specific malignancies such as lung cancer (SIR, 1.63; 95% CI, 1.43–1.87) and lymphoma (SIR, 2.08; 95% CI, 1.80–2.39) but a decreased risk of colorectal and breast cancer in patients with RA compared with the general population (**Table 1**).[16,19] Lymphoma was associated with the highest risk for malignancy, the pooled SIRs for lymphoma being 2.46 (95% CI, 2.05–2.96) with the risk of Hodgkin lymphoma (SIR, 3.21; 95% CI, 2.42–4.27) being numerically greater than that of non-Hodgkin lymphoma (SIR, 2.26; 95% CI, 1.82 to 2.81). There was no trend toward increased or decreased risk in RA for melanoma, cervical cancer, or prostate cancer.[19]

The impact of biologics on the risk of malignancies in patients with RA has been controversial. Some of the studies suggest increased risk,[18,23] whereas more recent population-based studies do not show any additional risk other than what already exists for patients with RA, noting the relationship of increased disease activity to development of lymphoid malignancy.[17,24] Data from various large European and US

Table 1
Pooled standardized incidence ratios for overall malignancies and site-specific malignancies in all patients with rheumatoid arthritis compared with the general population

Malignancy	Pooled Data, Studies (N)	Pooled SIRs (95% CI)
Overall	23	1.09 (1.06–1.13)
Lung cancer	23	1.64 (1.51–1.79)
Lymphoma	12	2.46 (2.05–2.96)
Hodgkin lymphoma	14	3.21 (2.42–4.27)
Non-Hodgkin lymphoma	17	2.26 (1.82–2.81)
Breast cancer	19	0.86 (0.73–1.01)
Colorectal cancer	23	0.78 (0.71–0.86)
Melanoma	21	1.23 (1.01–1.49)

SIR compared with SEER (US general population) data base.
Data from Simon TA, Thompson A, Gandhi KK. et al. Incidence of malignancy in adult patients with rheumatoid arthritis: a meta-analysis. Arthritis Res Ther 2015;17(1):212.

registry studies indicated that treatment of patients with RA with tumor necrosis factor (TNF) inhibitors is not associated with increased risks of non–skin cancer malignancies (odds ratio [OR], 0.95; 95% CI, 0.85–1.05), particularly lymphoma (OR = 1.1; 95% CI, 0.70–1.51) compared with treatment with traditional DMARDs.[21,25]

Protein tyrosine kinase inhibitors such as Jak inhibitors were originally developed for use in oncology. Imatinib, which is a protein tyrosine kinase inhibitor, has dramatically improved the outcomes for patients with chronic myelogenous leukemia, and other kinase inhibitors are used as treatment of renal cell carcinoma and small cell lung cancer. However, even though these therapies are used to treat cancer, concern over Jak inhibition and the significant impact on multiple cytokines with a potential for immunosuppression malignancy risk was a major issue monitored closely during the development program and postapproval for tofacitinib and more recently baricitinib. This article reviews the data available on malignancy risk and Jak inhibitor treatment of RA.

OVERALL MALIGNANCY IN PATIENTS WITH RHEUMATOID ARTHRITIS EXPOSED TO TOFACITINIB

Data assessing the risks of malignancies among JAK inhibitor users in RA are primarily obtained from individual randomized control trials (RCTs) and meta-analysis of RCTs. Although RCTs ensure comparability in the development of malignancies between the users and the placebo group, the short-term follow-up makes it difficult to quantify the exact incidence of malignancies in individuals using these medications. The ideal mechanism to obtain accurate data to assess the incidence of malignancies in JAK kinase inhibitors is the use of patient-based registries. However, JAK inhibitors in the treatment of RA have become available only recently, necessitating the use of RCTs to estimate the malignancy risk.

The bulk of the information on malignancy risk and tofacitinib is derived from the data presented to the FDA at the Arthritis Advisory Committee in 2012 and subsequent publications from the long-term extension (LTE) database of patients continuing on treatment following the randomized clinical trials. Approximately 4800 patients participated in the clinical trials on dosages of either 5 mg twice a day or 10 mg twice a day. The overall rates of malignancy in patients with RA receiving tofacitinib were similar to those of the general population and comparable with other biologics (**Figs. 1** and **2**, **Table 2**). There was concern that there was a trend for a higher risk for malignancy development in the LTE on the 10-mg dose compared with the 5-mg dose even though the rates were not statistically different except for the rate of NMSC in the LTE. At the Arthritis Advisory Committee meeting concern was expressed because of a modestly increased incidence of all malignancies (excluding NMSC) over time, with incidence rates of malignancies of 0.79 per 100 patient-years in the first 6 months with a peak incidence (1.93 per 100 patient-years) in 24 to 30 months. However, the number of subjects on treatment at the later time point was small compared with the earlier time points and an increased risk over time has not been reported with longer-term follow-up.[26,27]

In a recently published meta-analysis of 5671 patients with RA receiving tofacitinib in the phase 2/3 trials and LTE, a total of 107 patients (excluding patients with nonmelanoma cancers) developed malignancies. The most common malignancy was lung cancer (n = 24), followed by breast cancer (n = 19), lymphoma (n = 10), and gastric cancer (n = 6). Sixty-six patients developed nonmelanoma skin cancer, with a total of 82 nonmelanoma skin cancer (NMSC) events, including basal cell carcinoma (n = 44) and squamous cell cancer (n = 38). There were 18 deaths related to malignancies, with most being secondary to lung cancer (n = 10). The overall incidence rate (IR)

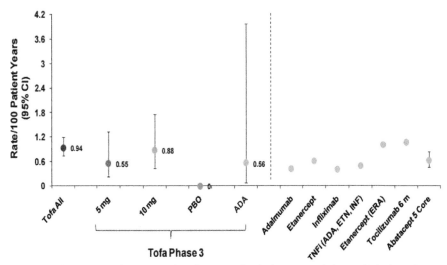

Fig. 1. Incidence rates (95% CI) of malignancy (excluding NMSC) from clinical trial data: tofacitinib (Tofa) versus TNF inhibitor and other biologic DMARDs. Malignancy, excluding NMSC. Bars indicate 95% confidence limits. Dots alone represent point estimates found in different published. ADA, adalimumab; ETN, etanercept; INF, infliximab; PBO, placebo; Tofa, tofacitinib. (*Adapted from* FDA Advisory Committee meeting briefing documents May 9th 2012. Available at: http://www.fda.gov/downloads/AdvisoryCommittees/Commit teesMeetingMaterials/Drugs/ArthritisAdvisoryCommittee/UCM302960.)

for all malignancies (excluding skin cancer) in patients with RA treated with tofacitinib was 0.85 (95% CI, 0.70–1.02). The incidences of all malignancy (excluding NMSC) were similar in the tofacitinib users compared with the general population (SIR, 1.17; 95% CI, 0.96–1.41). Patients on combination therapy (IR, 0.83; 95% CI, 0.53–1.28) had a numerically higher rate of malignancy compared with those on tofa- citinib monotherapy (IR, 0.32; 95% CI, 0.10–0.99), which was not statistically different.[27] There was no statistical difference in malignancy rates when stratified be- tween dose (5 mg vs 10 mg), duration of exposure to medication, and disease severity (moderate vs severe).[28–39]

Tofacitinib and Lung Cancer

The initial pooled data on the incidence of lung cancer from the RCTs and the LTE trials were reported by the FDA in 2012. A total of 16 cases (13 non–small cell cancer and 3 small cell cancer) were reported, with the overall incidence rates being 0.231 (95% CI, 0.142–0.377) per 100 patient-years of exposure. The reported SIR for all lung cancers compared with the general population was 2.35 (95% CI, 1.34–3.82).[26]

In the recent meta-analysis published in 2015, there were a total of 24 cases of lung cancer reported across all the phase 2, phase 3, and LTE trials. The overall IR was 0.19 (95% CI, 0.13–0.28) with an SIR of 2.19 (95% CI, 1.39–3.29) using the SEER for the comparator population. The presence of cancer was equally distributed among both genders. Patients taking higher doses of tofacitinib monotherapy (10 mg vs 5 mg) had a numerically higher rate of lung cancer (0.00; 95% CI, 0.00–0.82 vs 0.21; 95% CI, 0.03–1.52); however, there were no statistical differences in lung cancer between the two groups. The overall rates were stable over time. Use of DMARD at baseline in the tofacitinib group did not increase the risk of lung cancer compared with monotherapy.[27]

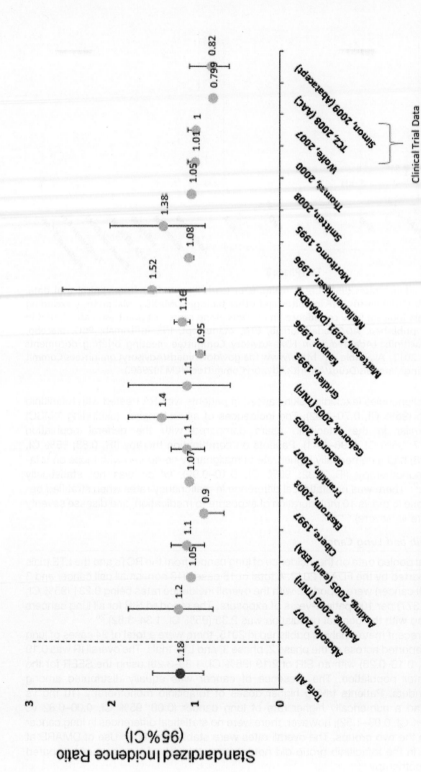

Fig. 2. SIRs (95% CI) for malignancy (excluding NMSC) from clinical trial data and observational data: tofacitinib versus TNF inhibitor and other biologic DMARDs. (*Adapted from* FDA Advisory Committee meeting briefing documents May 9th 2012. Available at: http://www.fda.gov/downloads/AdvisoryCommittees/CommitteesMeetingMaterials/Drugs/ArthritisAdvisoryCommittee/UCM302960)

Table 2
Standardized incidence ratios and incidence ratios for overall malignancies and site-specific malignancies for tofacitinib –treated patients with rheumatoid arthritis

Malignancy	Total Patients Tofacitinib (N)	SIRs (95% CI)	IR/100 Patient-Years (95% CI)
Overall (excluding NMSC)	5671	1.17 (0.96–1.41)	0.85 (0.70–1.02)
Lung cancer	5671	2.19 (1.39–3.29)	0.19 (0.13–0.28)
Lymphoma	5671	2.64 (1.27–4.86)	0.08 (0.04–0.14)
Breast cancer	5671	0.78 (0.47–1.22)	0.18 (0.12–0.28)
NMSC	5671	NR	0.53 (0.41–0.67)

SIR compared with SEER (US general population) data base.
Abbreviation: IR, incidence rate.
Adapted from Curtis JR, Lee EB, Kaplan IV, et al. Tofacitinib, an oral Janus kinase inhibitor: analysis of malignancies across the rheumatoid arthritis clinical development programme. Ann Rheum Dis 2015;75(5):1–11.

To place these data in perspective, the SIR of lung cancer for patients with RA receiving nonbiologic DMARDS compared with the general population is 2.39 (95% CI, 1.75–3.19), which is similar to that seen in patients receiving tofacitinib.[40] Similarly, use of biologics such as anti-TNF in RA has also shown a trend toward increase in risk for lung cancer compared with the general population (SIR, 1.8; 95% CI, 0.9–3.3).[41] Cigarette smoking is an independent risk factor for both RA and lung cancer and is the most important confounder in the assessment of RA and lung cancer risk. Seventy-five percent of the patients with RA treated with tofacitinib who developed lung cancer were either current (14 out of 24) or past smokers (6 out of 24), with a mean duration of 40 pack-years of smoking. Six out of 16 patients were diagnosed with lung cancer in the first 6 months of their treatment, suggesting that the cancer was present before entering the trial.[27] Overall, the risk of lung cancer in tofacitinib-treated patients, although increased compared with the general population, is similar to that seen in the overall RA population.

Tofacitinib and Lymphoma Risk

Lymphomas are a heterogeneous group of cancers arising from B and T cells.[42] These tumors result from chromosomal translocation, immunodeficiency subsets, certain environmental triggers, and chronic inflammation.[43] Malignant lymphomas, including Hodgkin lymphoma and non-Hodgkin lymphoma (NHL), account for approximately 4.8% of all cancers in the United States[22] and 4% to 5% of all cancers worldwide.[44,45] In 2015 alone 80,900 new cases of lymphoma were diagnosed, and the annual incidence rate of NHL is estimated to be 19.7 per 100,000 person years.[22] Certain autoimmune and chronic inflammatory states have been shown to have a higher lymphoma risk.[46,47]

The risk of development of lymphoma in patients with RA has been well established.[16,48] The reported relative risk (RR) for lymphoma in RA overall ranges from 1.5 to 4.0 with an average RR of 2.[16,46] The 2 most important risk factors for the development of lymphoma in RA are thought to be the presence of moderate to severe inflammation and the concomitant use of immunomodulators and biologics.[17,18,23] Although the correlation between severity of inflammation in RA and development of lymphoma has been well documented,[17] large cohort-based and registry-based studies have not been able to establish an association between lymphoma and use of DMARDs and biologics in RA.[17,21,49,50] Postmarketing surveillance data published by FDA reported the SIR of lymphoma in patients with RA to be as high as 5.4 in groups treated with adalimumab, 3.46 in groups treated with certolizumab, and 6.35 in groups treated with infliximab, suggesting a potential causal relationship.[26] In contrast, in a large US-based study of 13,001 patients with RA with 49,000 patient-years of exposure, the RR of lymphoma in the biologic treatment group was 1.7 compared with the general population, but the difference did not achieve statistical significance (OR, 1.0; 95% CI, 0.5–2.0).[21] In addition, in a cohort of the Swedish cancer registry of 6604 anti-TNF–treated patients with RA, compared with 2 comparator groups of anti-TNF–naive patients with RA and the general population, the risk of lymphoma in TNF-treated patients with RA was similar to that of TNF-naive patients with RA, with an RR of 1.35 (05% CI, 0.82–2.11), but higher than that of the general population, with an RR of 2.72 (95% CI, 1.82–4.08).[51]

In the development program for tofacitinib, a total of 10 cases of lymphoma were reported in patients with RA, 5 cases each in phase III and LTE trials.[33,36–39] There were no cases of lymphoma reported in phase II trials.[28–31] The overall IR was 0.08 per 100 patient-years (95% CI, 0.04–0.14). In the tofacitinib RCTs, the age-adjusted and sex-adjusted SIRs compared with the general population were 2.64 (95% CI, 1.27–4.86).[27] There were no reported cases of lymphoma in any of the placebo groups.[32,34,35]

The histology of lymphoma was heterogeneously distributed, with 8 of the 10 lymphoma being of the NHL type (including 1 large B-cell Burkitt type and 1 small B-cell mantle type), 90% of the cancers were the B-cell type, with just 1 patient having chronic T-cell lymphocytic leukemia.[27]

Lymphoma was reported in RCTs evaluating tofacitinib in renal transplant patients treated with other immunosuppressives and receiving higher doses of tofacitinib. The cause of posttransplant lymphoproliferative disorder (PTLD) after organ transplant is linked to the presence of Epstein-Barr virus (EBV) in the setting of immunosuppression.[52] The development of lymphomas was reported in 5 out of the 218 post–renal transplant patients (2.3%) receiving 15 mg of tofacitinib twice daily with other immunosuppressive drugs, including methylprednisolone, basiliximab, and mycophenolate mofetil. The incidence of PTLD in renal transplant patients on tofacitinib was higher then was expected in the general renal transplant population (0.55%–1%).[53,54] All 5 cases were associated with increased levels of EBV titers and higher tofacitinib blood concentration.[55] In patients with RA treated with tofacitinib, only 1 case of lymphoma had a positive EBV staining and there were 2 additional cases of equivocal EBV staining reported in patients receiving tofacitinib monotherapy. Unlike the association of EBV with PTLD in posttransplant immunosuppression patients, there are currently no conclusive data to link the use of tofacitinib with EBV-associated lymphomas in the nontransplant cohort of patients with RA.

In most tofacitinib trials, patients received either monotherapy or a combination with stably dosed DMARDs such as methotrexate. Patients receiving monotherapy with tofacitinib had similar rates of lymphoma compared with those receiving a combination of tofacitinib and methotrexate.[33,36–39]

Lymphomas were equally distributed among patients receiving 5 mg and 10 mg, with IRs of 0.08 (95% CI, 0.02–0.23) and 0.04 (95% CI, 0.01–0.15) respectively. The time to onset of lymphoma from initiation of treatment varied from as early as within 1 year of treatment (30%) to as late as 5 years (10%), with 80% of patients developing lymphoma in the first 2 years of treatment.[27] Even though 7 out of 10 patients who developed lymphoma were female, 80% of the subjects in the trial were female and the number of malignancies was too small to reach a conclusion about gender-based predilection to the development of RA in this cohort.

Based on the available data from the various tofacitinib RCTs and the LTE studies, it is apparent that the SIR for tofacitinib for lymphoma is comparable with that of patients with RA receiving nonbiologics and biologics, including anti-TNF.[16–19,21,26,33,36–39,51]

Nonmelanoma Skin Cancer

Basal cell carcinoma and squamous cell carcinoma are the 2 most common types of NMSC. A total 125 cases of NMSC was reported among 83 patients treated in all phase 1, phase 2, phase 3, and LTE studies. There were 51 cases of squamous cell cancer (n = 39), 71 cases of basal cell cancers (n = 52), and 11 patients with both squamous cell cancer and basal cell cancers. Most of the cancers were reported in the sun-exposed areas of the body, including hands, head, and face. The incidence of skin cancer was higher among white men and patients aged greater than 65 years. Patients receiving tofacitinib with background DMARDs had a similar IR of NMSC compared with tofacitinib monotherapy (0.64, 95% CI 0.49–0.84 vs 0. 43, 95% CI 0.30–0.64).[56] In a recent meta-analysis, the overall IR across phase 2, phase 3, and LTE trials for all NMSCs was 0.53 per 100 patient-years (95% CI, 0.41–6.7). In LTE trials the IR for NMSC was higher in the group receiving 10 mg (IR, 0.84; 95% CI, 0.62–1.13) compared with those receiving 5 mg (IR, 0.35; 95% CI, 0.21–0.51). The IR of NMSC was similar between the two dose groups in phase 3 trials. The development of skin cancers remained stable over time, with at least 10 cases developing within the first 6 months of exposure.[27]

Development of skin cancers in RA has been well reported to be increased compared with the general population. Data from epidemiologic studies have indicated an increased incidence of NMSC in treatment-naive patients with RA compared with the general population.[41,57–60] Among patients with RA, the development of NMSC is increased with use of steroids, anti-TNF alone, and/or with concomitant methotrexate use.[59] The use of biologics in RA was associated with increased risk of NMSC (OR, 1.5; 95% CI, 1.2–1.8) and melanoma (OR, 2.3; 95% CI, 0.9–5.4). Wolfe and colleagues[21] reported that TNF-treated patients with RA had an increased risk of NMSC (SIR, 1.5; 95% CI, 1.2–1.8) compared with the general population, which is similar to other published reports.[61] A recent publication confirmed the association of TNF inhibitors and increased risk of skin cancers, especially squamous cell cancer.[62]

The incident rates of skin cancers reported with biologic use in RA range from 0.17 to 1.81 events per 100 patient years observation[21,59,63] and are similar to those reported in patients with RA treated with tofacitinib.[27] In addition, the development of NMSC in tofacitinib was stable over time and possibly dose related, as suggested by the LTE data.

Breast Cancer

Breast cancer is the fourth most common cancer reported in clinical trials with tofacitinib. The malignancy data pooled from phase II, phase III, and LTE trials reported 19 cases of breast cancer among 5671 tofacitinib-treated patients and there were no cases reported in either the placebo or adalimumab groups, although exposure to these comparator groups was of short duration, making comparison difficult.[28–39] There was no difference in incidence of breast cancer among patients who received 10 mg of tofacitinib versus 5 mg in both phase III and LTE trials, and additionally the incidence was stable over time.[27] The SIR for breast cancer in patients with RA treated with TNF inhibitors and other biologic DMARDs ranges from 0.4 to 1.68 and is similar to that of tofacitinib.[16,21,26,27,41,64,65] Similarly, the incidence rates of breast cancer in tofacitinib-treated patients in RA (IR, 0.12–0.28 per 100 person-years) are consistent with published data among DMARD-treated and anti-TNF–treated (IR, 0.11–0.34 per 100 person-years) patients with RA.[26]

Other Cancers

Other malignancies reported in the phase 2, 3, and LTE program (**Table 3**) discussed earlier were gastric cancer (n = 7), prostate cancer (n = 6), colon cancer (n = 5), melanoma (n = 6), cervical cancer (n = 4), endometrial cancer (n = 4), ovarian cancer (n = 3), renal cancer (n = 3), thyroid cancer (n = 1), and unknown type (n = 16). No trend in development of malignancy was seen for tofacitinib.[27]

MORTALITY FROM MALIGNANCY

A total of 107 cases of malignancy (excluding NMSC) were reported from pooled data from 5671 patients, with 12,664 patient-years of exposure across all phase 2, 3, and LTE trials.[28–39] There were an additional 125 cases of NMSC reported in 83 patients in the tofacitinib RA trials.[56] A total of 18 deaths were reported in patients with RA treated with tofacitinib. Most of the deaths caused by malignancies were reported in patients with lung cancer (n = 10). There were 2 deaths from colon cancer and 1 each from malignancy related to breast, ovarian, colon, gastric hepatic, gallbladder, and synovial sarcoma. The number of deaths related to lung cancer was slightly higher in the 10-mg group (n = 7) compared with the 5-mg group (n = 3), but the overall mortality among all cancers was similar for both 5-mg and 10-mg doses of tofacitinib (8 vs 10 deaths, respectively).[27–39]

Table 3
Various malignancies in patients with rheumatoid arthritis treated with tofacitinib

Malignancy Type	Total Patients (N = 5671)
Cancers (excluding NMSC)	107
Lung cancer[a]	24
Breast cancer	19
Lymphoma/leukemia[b]	10
Gastric cancer	7
Prostate cancer	6
Melanoma	5
Colon cancer	5
Cervical cancer	4
Ovarian	4
Endometrial cancer	3
Renal cancer	3
Thyroid cancer	1
Unknown type	16
Nonmelanoma skin cancer	66

[a] Predominately non–small cell lung cancers.
[b] Non-Hodgkin lymphoma,[8] Hodgkin lymphoma,[1] and T-cell chronic lymphocytic leukemia.[1]
Data from Refs.[28–39]

OVERALL MALIGNANCY IN PATIENTS WITH RHEUMATOID ARTHRITIS EXPOSED TO BARICITINIB

At present there are 2 published phase 2 and 1 phase 3 placebo-controlled clinical trials evaluating the efficacy and safety of baricitinib in active RA (N = 973). There were just 2 reported cases of NMSC and none of the patients developed solid tumors in either of the studies.[6,66–68] More recently, a novel JAK-1 inhibitor (ABT-494) is being investigated (phase 2b) in TNF-intolerant patients with RA, with no reported cases of solid organ tumors.[56,58]

SUMMARY

The use of biologics such as anti-TNF and, more recently, the availability of oral Jak inhibitors such as tofacitinib have revolutionized the management and treatment of RA. Because of the mechanism of action of the Jak inhibitors, concern over the risk of malignancies related to immunosuppression exist, similar to previous concerns after the introduction of the biologics. Based on the RCT and LTE data, the risk of malignancy with tofacitinib 5 mg twice a day is similar to that seen with biologics. Similar to biologics, an increased risk for certain site-specific malignancies, including lung cancer, lymphoma, and NMSC, compared with the general population was noted.[17–19,21,23,27,51] There was a trend for an increased risk of malignancies with the 10-mg dose, which has not been approved in the United States, but the difference was not statistically significant except for NMSCs. In addition, the rate of malignancies did not increase over time in the LTE observational cohort. At present there are insufficient data linking baricitinib with development of malignancies, and results from LTE are awaited.[6,66,67]

Additional results from the LTE will soon be available, along with information on patients enrolled in prospective observational registries. Based on the limited data on 5671 patients with 12,664 patient-years of exposure, health care providers and patients should be comfortable that the risk of malignancy associated with tofacitinib and, to a lesser degree, baricitinib is similar to that associated with biologics. As with biologics, for which limited data are available, the risk of Jak inhibitors for recurrent cancer in patients with previous malignancy is unknown because these patients were excluded from the RCTs.

REFERENCES

1. Hoes JN, Jacobs JW, Verstappen SM, et al. Adverse events of low to medium dose oral glucocorticoids in inflammatory diseases: a meta-analysis. Ann Rheum Dis 2009;68:1833–8.
2. Fortunet C, Pers YM, Lambert J, et al. Tocilizumab induces corticosteroid sparing in rheumatoid arthritis patients in clinical practice. Rheumatology (Oxford) 2015; 54(4):672–7.
3. Seror R, Dougados M, Gossec L. Glucocorticoid sparing effect of tumour necrosis factor alpha inhibitors in rheumatoid arthritis in real life practice. Clin Exp Rheumatol 2009;27(5):807–13.
4. Navmann L, Huscher D, Detert J, et al. Anti tumour necrosis factor alpha therapy in patients with rheumatoid arthritis results in a significant and long lasting decrease of concomitant glucocorticoid treatment. Ann Rheum Dis 2009; 68(12):1934–6.
5. Mavers M, Ruderman E, Perlman H. Intracellular signal pathways: potential for therapies. Curr Rheumatol Rep 2009;11(5):378–85.

6. Genovese MC, Kremer J, Zamani O, et al. Baricitinib in patients with refractory rheumatoid arthritis. N Engl J Med 2016;374(13):1243–52.

7. Darnell JE, Kerr I, Stark G. Jak-STAT pathways and transcriptional activation in response to IFNs and other extracellular signaling proteins. Science 1994;264: 1415–21.

8. Pesu M, Candotti F, Husa M, et al. Jak 3, severe combined immunodeficiency, and a new class of immunosuppressive drugs. Immunol Rev 2005;203:127–42.

9. Ghoreschi K, Jesson M, Li X, et al. Modulation of innate and adaptive immune responses by tofacitinib. J Immunol 2011;186(7):4234–43.

10. Levine RL, Wadleigh M, Cools J, et al. Activating mutation in the tyrosine kinase Jak 2 in polycythemia vera, essential thrombocythemia, and myeloid metaplasia with myelofibrosis. Cancer Cell 2005;7:387–97.

11. Harrison C, Kiladjian J, Al-Ali H, et al. JAK inhibition with ruxolitinib versus best available therapy for myelofibrosis. New Eng J Med 2012;366(9):787–98.

12. Tokumasa N, Suto A, Kagami S, et al. Expression of Tyk 2 in dendritic cells is required for IL-12, IL-23, and IFN-gamma production and the induction of TH1 cell differentiation. Blood 2007;110:553–60.

13. Kubler K. Janus kinase inhibitors: mechanisms of action. Aust Prescr 2014;37: 154–7.

14. Hodge JA, Kawabata TT, Krishnaswami S, et al. The mechanism of action of tofacitinib – an oral Janus kinase inhibitor for the treatment of rheumatoid arthritis. Clin Exp Rheumatol 2016;34(2):318–28.

15. Singh J, Saag K, Bridges L, et al. 2015 American College of Rheumatology guideline for the treatment of rheumatoid arthritis. Arthritis Care Res (Hoboken) 2016;68(1):1–25.

16. Smitten A, Simon T, Hochberg M. A meta-analysis of the incidence of malignancy in adult patients with rheumatoid arthritis. Arthritis Res Ther 2008;10:R45.

17. Baecklund E, Iliadou A, Askling J. Association of chronic inflammation, not its treatment, with increased lymphoma risk in rheumatoid arthritis. Arthritis Rheum 2006;54:692–701.

18. Bongartz T, Sutton AJ, Sweeting MJ. Anti TNF antibody therapy in rheumatoid arthritis and the risk of serious infections and malignancies. Systemic review and meta-analysis of rare harmful effects in randomized controlled trials. JAMA 2006;295:2275–85.

19. Simon TA, Thompson A, Gandhi KK, et al. Incidence of malignancy in adult patients with rheumatoid arthritis: a meta-analysis. Arthritis Res Ther 2015;17(1): 212.

20. Chakravarthy EF, Genovesse MC. Association between rheumatoid arthritis and malignancy. Rheum Dis Clin North Am 2004;30:271–84.

21. Wolfe F, Michaud K. Biologic treatment of rheumatoid arthritis and the risk of malignancy: analyses from a large US observational study. Arthritis Rheum 2007;56: 2886–9.

22. National Cancer Institute. Surveillance, epidemiology and end results. Available at: http://seer.cancer.gov/.

23. Wolfe F, Michaud K. Lymphoma in rheumatoid arthritis: the effect of methotrexate and anti tumour necrosis factor therapy in 18,572 patients. Arthritis Rheum 2004; 50:1740–51.

24. Olivo L, Tayar JH. Risk of malignancies in patients with rheumatoid arthritis treated with biologic therapy. A meta-analysis. JAMA 2012;308:898–908.

25. Codreanu C, Damjanov N. Safety of biologics in rheumatoid arthritis: data from randomized controlled trials and registries. Biologics 2015;9:1–6.

26. FDA Advisory Committee meeting briefing documents, FDA white Oak conference center, Maryland, May 9th, 2012.

27. Curtis JR, Lee EB, Kaplan IV, et al. Tofacitinib, an oral Janus kinase inhibitor: analysis of malignancies across the rheumatoid arthritis clinical development programme. Ann Rheum Dis 2016;75(5):831–41.

28. Kremer JM, Bloom BJ, Breedveld FC, et al. The safety and efficacy of a JAK inhibitor in patients with active rheumatoid arthritis: results of a double blind, placebo-controlled phase IIa trial of three dosage levels of CP-690,550 versus placebo. Arthritis Rheum 2009;60:1895–905.

29. Fleischmann R, Cutolo M, Genovese MC, et al. Phase IIb dose-ranging study of the oral JAK inhibitor tofacitinib or adalimumab monotherapy versus placebo in patients with active rheumatoid arthritis with an inadequate response to disease modifying antirheumatic drugs. Arthritis Rheum 2012;64:617–29.

30. Tanaka Y, Takeuchi T, Yamanaka H, et al. Efficacy and safety of tofacitinib as monotherapy in Japanese patients with active rheumatoid arthritis: a 12-week, randomized, phase 2 study. Mod Rheumatol 2015;25(4):514–21.

31. Kremer JM, Cohen S, Wilkinson BE, et al. A phase IIb dose-ranging study of the oral JAK inhibitor tofacitinib (CP-690,550) versus placebo in combination with background methotrexate in patients with active rheumatoid arthritis and an inadequate response to methotrexate alone. Arthritis Rheum 2012;64:970–81.

32. Burmester GR, Blanco R, Charles-Schoeman C, et al. Tofacitinib (CP-690,550) in combination with methotrexate in patients with active rheumatoid arthritis with an inadequate response to tumor necrosis factor inhibitors: a randomized phase 3 Trial. Lancet 2013;381:451–60.

33. Lee EB, Fleischmann R, Hall S, et al. Tofacitinib versus methotrexate in rheumatoid arthritis. N Engl J Med 2014;370:2377–86.

34. Kremer J, Li ZG, Hall S, et al. Tofacitinib in combination with nonbiologic DMARDs in patients with active rheumatoid arthritis: a randomized trial. Ann Intern Med 2013;159:253–61.

35. Fleischmann R, Kremer J, Cush J, et al. Placebo-controlled trial of tofacitinib monotherapy in rheumatoid arthritis. N Engl J Med 2012;367:495–507.

36. Vollenhoven V, Fleischmann R, Cohen S, et al. Tofacitinib or adalimumab versus placebo in rheumatoid arthritis. N Engl J Med 2012;367:508–19.

37. Van der Heijde D, Tanaka Y, Fleischmann R, et al. Tofacitinib in patients with rheumatoid arthritis receiving methotrexate: twelve-month data from twenty four month phase III randomized radiographic study. Arthritis Rheum 2013;65:559–70.

38. Wollenhaupt J, Silverfield J, Lee EB, et al. Safety and efficacy of tofacitinib, an oral Janus kinase inhibitor, for the treatment of rheumatoid arthritis in open label, long term extension studies. J Rheumatol 2014;41:837–52.

39. Yamanaka H, Tanaka Y, Takeuchi T, et al. Tofacitinib an oral Janus kinase inhibitor, as monotherapy or with background methotrexate in Japanese patients with rheumatoid arthritis: a phase 2/3 long-term extension study. Arthritis Rheum 2011;63:1215 [abstract: S473].

40. Mercer LK, Galloway DR, Dixon L, et al. Risk of cancer in patients receiving nonbiologic disease modifying therapy for rheumatoid arthritis compared with the UK general population. Rheumatology (Oxford) 2013;52:91–8.

41. Askling J, Fored CM, Brandt L, et al. Risks of solid cancers in patients with rheumatoid arthritis and after treatment with tumor necrosis factor antagonists. Ann Rheum Dis 2005;64:1421–6.

42. Kippers R. Hodgkin's lymphoma. J Clin Invest 2012;122:3439–47.

43. Vose JM. Peripheral T cell non-Hodgkin's lymphoma. Hematol Oncol Clin North Am 2008;22(5):997–1005.
44. Sandin S. Incidence of non-Hodgkin's lymphoma in Sweden, Denmark, and Finland from 1960 through 2003: an epidemic that was. Cancer Epidemiol biomarkers prev 2006;15:1295–300.
45. Chang KC, Huang GC, Jones D, et al. Distribution and prognosis of WHO lymphoma subtypes in Taiwan reveals a low incidence of germinal-center derived tumors. Leuk Lymphoma 2004;45:1375–84.
46. Zintzaras E. Risk of lymphoma development in autoimmune diseases: a meta-analysis. Arch Intern Med 2005;165:2337–44.
47. Ekstrom K, Hjalgrim H, Brandt L, et al. Risk of malignant lymphomas in patients with rheumatoid arthritis and in their first-degree relatives. Arthritis Rheum 2003;48:963–70.
48. Baecklund E, Askling J, Rosenquist R, et al. Rheumatoid arthritis and malignant lymphomas. Curr Opin Rheumatol 2004;16:254–61.
49. Mariette X, Cazals-Hatem D, Warszawki J, et al. Lymphomas in rheumatoid arthritis patients treated with methotrexate: a 3-year prospective study in France. Blood 2002;99(11):3909–15.
50. Dematsky S, Clarke AE, Suissa S. Hematologic malignant neoplasms after drug exposure in rheumatoid arthritis. Arch Intern Med 2008;168(4):378–81.
51. Askling J, Baecklund E, Granath F, et al. Anti-tumour necrosis factor therapy in rheumatoid arthritis and risk of malignant lymphomas: relative risks and time trends in the Swedish Biologics Register. Ann Rheum Dis 2009;68(5):648–53.
52. Taylor AL, Marcus R, Bradley AJ. Post-transplant lymphoproliferative disorders (PTLD) after solid organ transplantation. Crit Rev Oncol Hematol 2005;56(1): 155–67.
53. Caillard S, Dharnidharka V, Agodoa L, et al. Post transplant lymphoproliferative disorders after renal transplantation in the United States in era of modern immunosuppression. Transplantation 2005;80(9):1233–43.
54. Caillard S, Lelong C, Pessione F, et al. Post-transplant lymphoproliferative disorders occurring after renal transplantation in adults: report of 230 cases from the French Registry. Am J Transplant 2006;6(11):2735–42.
55. Vincenti F, Silva TH, Busque SO, et al. Randomized phase 2b trial of tofacitinib (CP-690,550) in de novo kidney transplant patients: efficacy, renal function and safety at 1 year. Am J Transplant 2012;12:2446–56.
56. Curtis JR, Lee EB, Martin G, et al. Analysis of non-melanoma skin cancer across the tofacitinib rheumatoid arthritis clinical program, 16th annual European congress of rheumatology, Rome (Italy), June 10-13, 2015.
57. Gridley G, Mclaughlin JK, Ekbom A, et al. Incidence of cancer among patients with rheumatoid arthritis. J Natl Cancer Inst 1993;85:307–11.
58. Mellemkjaer L, Linet MS, Gridley G, et al. Rheumatoid arthritis and cancer risk. Eur J Cancer 1996;32A:1753–7.
59. Chakravarty EF, Michaud K, Wolfe F. Skin cancer, rheumatoid arthritis and tumor necrosis factor inhibitors. J Rheumatol 2005;32:2130–5.
60. Dreyer L, Mellemkjaer L, Anderson AR, et al. Incidence of overall and site specific cancers in TNF alpha inhibitor treated patients with rheumatoid arthritis and other arthritides–a follow up study from the DANBIO Registry. Ann Rheum Dis 2013;72: 79–82.
61. Moulis G, Sommet A, Bene J, et al. Cancer risk and Anti TNF alpha at recommended doses in adult rheumatoid arthritis: a meta analysis with intention to treat and per protocol analyses. PLoS One 2012;7:e48991.

62. Raaschou P. Rheumatoid arthritis, anti-tumour necrosis factor treatment and risk of squamous cell and basal cell skin cancer: cohort study based on nationwide prospectively recorded data from Sweden. BMJ 2016;352:i262.
63. Askling J, Fahrbach K, Nordstrom B, et al. Cancer risk with tumor necrosis factor alpha (TNF) inhibitors: meta-analysis of randomized controlled trials of adalimumab, etanercept, and infliximab using patient level data. Pharmacoepidemiol Drug Saf 2011;20:119–30.
64. Abasolo L, Judez E, Descalzo M, et al. Cancer in rheumatoid arthritis: occurrence, mortality, and associated factors in a south European population. Semin Arthritis Rheum 2008;37:388–97.
65. Setoguchi S, Solomon DH, Weinblatt ME, et al. Tumor necrosis factor alpha antagonist use and cancer in patients with rheumatoid arthritis. Arthritis Rheum 2006;54:2757–64.
66. Keystone E, Emery P, Camp H, et al. Safety and efficacy of baricitinib at 24 weeks in patients with rheumatoid arthritis who have had an inadequate response to methotrexate. Ann Rheum Dis 2015;74:333–40.
67. Tanaka Y, Emoto K, Cai Z, et al. Efficacy and safety of baricitinib in Japanese patients with active rheumatoid arthritis receiving background methotrexate therapy: a 12 week, double blind, randomized placebo controlled study. J Rheumatol 2016; 43(3):504–11.
68. Kremer JM, Keystone EC, Emery P, et al. Selective Jak 1 inhibitor in patients with active rheumatoid arthritis and inadequate response or intolerance to anti-TNF biologic therapy. 2015 ACR/ARHP Annual Meeting. [abstract: 14L].

The Risk of Progressive Multifocal Leukoencephalopathy in the Biologic Era
Prevention and Management

Eamonn S. Molloy, MD, MS, FRCPI[a],*, Cassandra M. Calabrese, DO[b],
Leonard H. Calabrese, DO[b]

KEYWORDS

- Progressive multifocal leukoencephalopathy • Biologic therapy
- Synthetic immunosuppressive therapy • Autoimmune rheumatic diseases
- Systemic lupus erythematosus • Rituximab

KEY POINTS

- Progressive multifocal leukoencephalopathy (PML) is a frequently fatal demyelinating infection of the central nervous system due to reactivation of the ubiquitous John Cunningham polyomavirus in immunosuppressed patients.
- PML has been reported in patients with rheumatic disease, with a disproportionate occurrence in systemic lupus erythematosus.
- A variety of rheumatic disease therapies have been associated with PML, with a disproportionate signal for rituximab. In a notable minority of patients, PML occurs in the setting of minimal iatrogenic immunosuppression.
- Increased awareness of PML is necessary, as early diagnosis and withdrawal of immunosuppressive therapy may improve outcomes.

INTRODUCTION

Progressive multifocal leukoencephalopathy (PML) is a rare, central nervous system (CNS) demyelinating disease that occurs predominantly in immunosuppressed patient populations. The etiologic agent is the John Cunningham virus (JCV),[1] a polyomavirus that is widely distributed in the form of a latent infection in the general population. In the setting of PML, JCV becomes activated leading to infection and destruction of myelin-producing oligodendrocytes. PML is typically fatal; most survivors have

Disclosures: None.
[a] Department of Rheumatology, St Vincent's University Hospital, Elm Park, Dublin 4, Ireland;
[b] RJ Fasenmeyer Center for Clinical Immunology, Department of Rheumatic and Immunologic Diseases, Cleveland Clinic, 9500 Euclid Avenue, Cleveland, OH 44195, USA
* Corresponding author.
E-mail address: e.molloy@svuh.ie

Rheum Dis Clin N Am 43 (2017) 95–109
http://dx.doi.org/10.1016/j.rdc.2016.09.009
rheumatic.theclinics.com

devastating neurologic sequelae. These poor outcomes are compounded by the lack of a proven effective antiviral therapy.

Although PML has in recent decades been described predominantly in patients infected with the human immunodeficiency virus (HIV), it is also well recognized in other immunosuppressed patient populations including those with malignancies and organ transplants. PML has recently attracted the attention of specialists treating patients with various autoimmune diseases, following reports of its association with the use of a number of immunosuppressive therapies, such as natalizumab, efalizumab, mycophenolate mofetil, and rituximab. Although all patients with rheumatic disease, regardless of the intensity of their current immunosuppressive therapy, should be considered potentially at risk of PML, informed clinical decision-making requires understanding the risk of PML associated with these therapies and the underlying autoimmune disease.

This article reviews the pathogenesis, clinical features and diagnosis of PML, summarizes the available evidence regarding the risk of PML associated with rheumatic diseases and relevant therapies, and highlights the dearth of effective preventive and management strategies for PML in this setting.

PATHOGENESIS
John Cunningham Virus Infection

The etiologic agent for PML, the human polyoma virus JC, is among a growing list of human pathogens of this genus, the most common of which are JC, BK (responsible for nephropathy in the immunosuppressed), and Merkel cell polyoma virus (associated with Merkel cell carcinoma of the skin).[2,3] JCV is ubiquitously found in virtually all sources of sewage, and although unproven is presumed to be spread in late childhood via an oral or respiratory route, although no primary clinical syndrome has been described. Seroepidemiologic evidence suggests more than half of the adult population is infected.[3] In healthy adults, the infection is lifelong, which results in periodic viral shedding in the urine from host resident tissue in the kidneys. Other tissues, such as bone marrow, may be seeded but viremia is extremely rare.[3,4] Whether seeding of the CNS occurs early or only after reactivation is controversial, but recent studies suggest asymptomatic infection on CNS tissues occurs more commonly that previously suspected[5] and is increased in immunosuppressed individuals in the absence of PML.[6,7]

Development of Progressive Multifocal Leukoencephalopathy

The rarity of PML compared with the ubiquitous nature of JCV infection indicates that there are likely multiple strong barriers to the development of PML.[8] Consensus exists that there are 3 barriers to the development of disease, including host factors, viral factors, and immunologic barriers. Host factors remain the most speculative of these, but viral and immunologic factors are becoming better understood.

Host factors

As long as the host's immune system is intact, JC infection does not cause PML. In contrast, during periods of immunocompromise there are subsequent changes in viral structure and cellular tropism that allow propagation of the infection in the CNS. JCV infects primarily myelin-producing oligodendrocytes as well as astrocytes, resulting in PML. PML may arise in primary states of immunosuppression, such as in primary CD4 lymphopenia,[4,9] but is observed far more commonly in acquired states of immunodeficiency, such as HIV, which still accounts for nearly 80% of all cases.[4] Rarely patients with minimal or no detectable immune deficiency states develop the disease.[10] Of particular interest to rheumatologists is the increasing recognition that iatrogenic immunosuppression with conventional immunosuppressives, such as mycophenolate and cyclophosphamide, and, more recently, biologic agents, such as rituximab and belimumab, all may contribute to the development of PML.[11–14]

Viral factors

A critical stage in the evolution of PML is a change in viral structure, primarily in its regulatory region as well as possibly in at least one of its outer capsid proteins. This structural change marks a shift from the wild type known as *archetype* to an altered form displaying neurotropism often referred to as *prototype* virus.[1,5] How exactly JCV shifts from its latent repositories of renal tissue and bone marrow and when this occurs are still poorly understood. JCV may occur as free virions in blood but also may be cell-associated; there is evidence of infection of virtually all subpopulations[3] and in particular B cells.[15] A schematic of JC viral infection and immunopathogenesis is displayed in **Fig. 1**. There are still gaping holes in our knowledge of JCV immunopathogenesis, including how and when the virus extends to the CNS and which aspects of the integrated immune system are dominant in ultimate control of viral changes leading to transformation into its neurotropic form.

Immune factors

Multiple lines of evidence suggest that PML results frequently if not exclusively from viral reactivation and not newly acquired infection. These data include the paucity of disease is seen in children and recent data from patients developing PML in the setting of natalizumab confirming the presence of virus 6 to 180 months before disease onset.[16] Evidence for a prominent role of suppressed immunity and in particular cell-mediated immunity include its clinical rarity in healthy individuals and its strong association with disease affecting T-cell–mediated immunity, especially HIV disease, as well as lymphoproliferative diseases and immunosuppressive therapies. Furthermore,

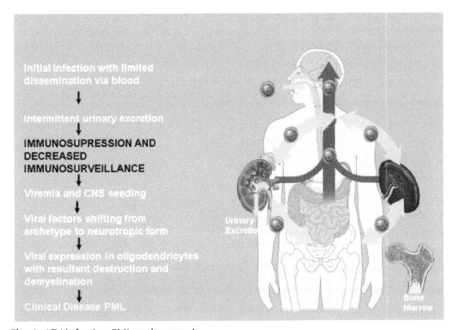

Fig. 1. JCV infection PML pathogenesis.

survival from PML has been documented in substantial numbers of people when the immune system has been restored.[17]

The immunopathology of PML is classically characterized by a notable lack of inflammation in the pathologic lesions, which correlates with the characteristic lack of contrast enhancement on gadolinium-enhanced MRI. This is in line with a model of disease resulting from progressive degradation of integrated host defense against the virus.[1,18] More recently (primarily in the context of PML associated with iatrogenic immunosuppression or that recognized in the wake of robust immune reconstitution, as seen in patients with HIV treated with combination antiretrovirals), an immune reconstitution syndrome pathologically characterized by a massive influx of inflammatory cells has been well-described. Clinically, such patients may deteriorate from expanding pathologic lesions attended by mass effect and often, but not always, associated with contrast enhancement on MRI.[17] Awareness of this syndrome is critical to effective management, as now 70% to 80% of such patients can survive with effective immune reconstitution.[17]

DIAGNOSIS

Diagnosis of PML requires history and physical examination findings suggestive of PML, characteristic MRI findings, and demonstration of JCV (typically JCV DNA in the cerebrospinal fluid [CSF]) (**Box 1**).[4] When considering a diagnosis of PML, there are many differential diagnoses that must first be excluded. These include infections such as herpes simplex encephalitis, varicella-zoster virus encephalopathy, and HIV encephalopathy. Noninfectious etiologies include CNS lymphoma, reversible posterior leukoencephalopathy, and CNS manifestations of systemic rheumatic diseases.

Clinical Features

The signs and symptoms of PML are highly variable and depend on the area of brain involved. Demyelination most commonly occurs in the subcortical white matter of the cerebral hemispheres, cerebellum, or brainstem. The clinical presentation is characterized by focal neurologic deficits that are insidious in onset and follow a progressive

---

Box 1
Diagnosis of progressive multifocal leukoencephalopathy

Clinical Features

- Subacute onset of neurologic deficits
- Absence of optic nerve involvement
- Absence of spinal cord disease

MRI features

- Unifocal or multifocal lesions of the white matter
- Lesions are typically nonenhancing
- Lesions lack mass effect

Polymerase Chain Reaction Analysis

- John Cunningham virus DNA detectable in cerebrospinal fluid (or in brain biopsy)

Adapted from Brew BJ, Davies NW, Cinque P, et al. Progressive multifocal leukoencephalopathy and other forms of JC virus disease. Nat Rev Neurol 2010;6:667–79.

course. In general, presenting symptoms include cognitive dysfunction, motor deficits, aphasia, ataxia, and visual symptoms, most commonly hemianopia and diplopia.[1] Seizures are a presenting feature in up to 18% of patients.[19] The spinal cord and optic nerve are virtually never affected and their involvement should suggest an alternative diagnosis.

Laboratory Testing

There are no routine laboratory tests that can confirm or rule out the diagnosis of PML. JCV DNA is detected in plasma in a very small percentage of randomly selected healthy individuals; this frequency is elevated in some high-risk populations (eg, HIV-infected subjects). JCV-specific antibodies are detectable in at least half of the general population. However, neither test is of diagnostic value for PML. All patients with suspected PML require laboratory evaluation for other potential causes, in particular HIV infection.

Radiology

Imaging plays an important role in the diagnostic and prognostic evaluation of PML. Computed tomography imaging of the brain may reveal hypodense, nonenhancing lesions in the white matter; however, MRI is the most sensitive imaging modality to detect lesions of PML.[20] Typical MRI findings include asymmetrical subcortical hyperintensities on T2-weighted and fluid-attenuated inversion recovery (FLAIR) sequences (**Fig. 2**). Changes are hypointense on T1-weighted imaging. Supratentorial lesions are more common than brainstem and/or cerebellar involvement. Thalamic and/or basal ganglia involvement is less common, but has been reported.[21,22] Cortical gray matter can be involved in a secondary fashion in up to one-quarter of patients with PML; it is presumed to be due to U-fiber involvement at the gray-white matter interface.[23]

Mass effect and contrast enhancement are not common findings; however, in certain cases such as in the setting of biologic therapies or immune reconstitution syndrome in HIV infection, inflammatory PML lesions can be seen and complicate the diagnosis.[24] Inflammatory PML lesions enhance on T1-weighted scans following gadolinium administration. The presence of enhancing PML lesions on brain MRI in patients with HIV+ PML treated with highly active antiretroviral therapy (HAART) correlates with better prognosis.

Cerebrospinal Fluid Analysis

CSF analysis is critical in the evaluation of patients with suspected PML not only to secure the diagnosis of PML but also from the perspective of excluding other diagnoses. Routine CSF analysis is typically nondescript with normal/mild elevations of CSF cell count and protein. Detecting JCV by polymerase chain reaction (PCR) in the CSF is the critical test for diagnosis of PML; this has a reported sensitivity of 72% to 92% and specificity approaching 100% in the pre-HAART era.[25] Therefore, detection of JCV in the CSF is essentially diagnostic for PML, but negative results do not exclude PML.

Brain Biopsy

Brain biopsy is the most specific diagnostic modality but is rarely required. Biopsy should be considered if clinical suspicion for PML is high and PCR of the CSF is repeatedly negative. Typical findings include extensive demyelination; oligodendroglia with enlarged, glassy nuclei characteristic of viral inclusion bodies; atypical reactive astrocytes of variable morphology; and a variable degree of lymphocytic inflammatory response. The inflammatory infiltration in PML has been historically described as

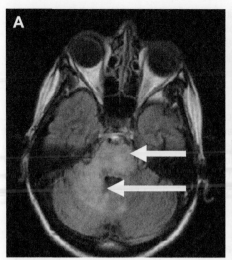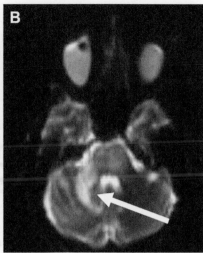

Fig. 2. A 42-year-old woman with a 27 year history of SLE, treated with hydroxychloroquine, presented to an outside hospital with a 1-month history of cerebellar symptoms; nonenhancing white matter lesions in the right cerebellar hemisphere and brachium pontis were noted on MRI. CSF cell count and biochemical analysis were within normal limits. She was diagnosed with lupus cerebritis, and treated with high-dose glucocorticoids. She subsequently developed progressive neurologic symptoms with left-sided sensory disturbance, mood disorder, and mycophenolate mofetil was added. One month after her initial presentation, she was admitted to the Cleveland Clinic. MRI brain and repeat CSF analysis were performed. FLAIR images (*A*) showed lesions (*arrows*) with increased signal affecting pons and right cerebellum; corresponding lesions (*arrow*) were seen on diffusion-weighted images (*B*). Routine CSF analysis was normal. After initial aggressive treatment for presumed lupus cerebritis was instituted with intravenous cyclophosphamide and methylprednisolone, CSF PCR testing for JCV was reported to be positive. A diagnosis of PML was made on the basis of progressive neurologic decline during immunosuppressive therapy, the compatible neuroimaging, and CSF findings. Immunosuppressive therapy was withdrawn. No specific antiviral treatment was instituted and the patient died shortly thereafter, approximately 3 months after her initial presentation with neurologic symptoms.

containing almost exclusively foamy macrophages with sparse lymphocytic reaction. However, PML cases with intense CNS lymphocytic infiltration have been frequently reported during the HAART era,[24,26,27] in non-HIV[24] cases, and in cases with discontinuation of immunosuppressant[28] or without obvious underlying immune disorder.[22] Evidence of the presence of JCV should be sought by immunohistochemistry (IHC), in situ hybridization, and/or PCR. IHC may have suboptimal sensitivity and therefore should be combined with another technique.[29]

PROGRESSIVE MULTIFOCAL LEUKOENCEPHALOPATHY AND THE RHEUMATOLOGIST

PML is of relevance to rheumatologists for a number of reasons. First, as described in a survey of rheumatologists' knowledge of and attitudes toward PML, concerns over PML significantly affect patients' and physicians' decisions on the choice of immunosuppressive therapies.[30] Second, with the recognition of a possible inflammatory component to PML, as described previously, it is clear that PML may closely mimic the neuroinflammatory manifestations of autoimmune rheumatic diseases. Third,

PML is likely underdiagnosed in patients with autoimmune rheumatic diseases, as the diagnosis of PML may not be considered initially in patients that succumb to presumed autoimmune neuroinflammatory manifestations of rheumatic disease.[31] Further, rheumatologists have important real and perceived learning gaps regarding PML; for example, 41% of those surveyed could not identify the diagnostic test of choice for PML.[30]

Differentiating PML from the new onset or exacerbation of CNS complications of various rheumatic diseases can be problematic, as exemplified by the case outlined in **Fig. 2**. Diagnostic difficulties are particularly salient for acute neuropsychiatric systemic lupus erythematosus (SLE) and vasculitis affecting the CNS. Underscoring the importance of differentiating PML from these conditions is that initiating or escalating immunosuppressive therapy, which is beneficial in immune-mediated CNS disease, is diametrically opposite of the treatment strategy for PML, which is to restore host defenses to the extent possible.

Clinical history and examination remain an important discriminator between PML and neuropsychiatric SLE or CNS vasculitis. Involvement of optic nerve or spinal cord is extremely rare in PML and argues strongly against this diagnosis. Subacute symptom evolution with rapid and relentless progression typifies PML. MRI brain may be suggestive, but does not provide unambiguous distinction between these uncommon conditions. It is relatively straightforward to differentiate PML from CNS vasculitis when there is evidence of multifocal cerebral ischemia and infarction of both gray and white matter, as infarction does not occur in PML. Unfortunately, MR imaging in both PML and CNS vasculitis can be nonspecific, with the latter occasionally showing foci of T2 hyperintensity occurring predominantly in the white matter[32,33] or even more rarely when found exclusively and diffusely in the white matter.[34] Angiography, although normal in PML, also may be normal in CNS vasculitis with small vessel involvement.

CSF analysis is critical in assessing the presence of JCV (and other opportunistic pathogens) in suspected neuropsychiatric SLE or CNS vasculitis with atypical features or when the patient unexpectedly worsens despite intensive immunosuppressive therapy. Detection of JCV in the CSF is diagnostic for PML, but negative results do not exclude PML. Acute neuropsychiatric SLE may be even more challenging to differentiate from PML when neuroimaging abnormalities are limited to the white matter in a patient deteriorating neurologically on immunosuppressive therapy. CSF analysis may be unhelpful in determining if SLE is responsible for the clinical picture, given that it may be normal in up to 50% of patients with neuropsychiatric SLE. The presence of enhancement following gadolinium administration, which is common in acute neuropsychiatric SLE, was once thought to be absent in PML, but is well-described in PML in a variety of disease settings, as discussed previously. Therefore, differentiating PML from other conditions is difficult based on the observation of enhancing CNS lesions alone. When evidence of frank infarction is present, such findings favor vasculitis or SLE.[35] Given that PML and CNS complications from any rheumatic disease may coexist, it appears prudent to consider this complication whenever the clinical situation warrants and to pursue the diagnosis with CSF analysis for the presence of JCV, and CNS biopsy if necessary.

PROGRESSIVE MULTIFOCAL LEUKOENCEPHALOPATHY IN RHEUMATIC DISEASES
Contribution of Underlying Rheumatic Disease

The Food and Drug Administration (FDA) issued an alert in December 2006 following documentation of 2 fatal cases of PML in patients with SLE, both of whom had been treated with rituximab.[36] We subsequently performed a search of the English-language medical literature to identify cases of PML associated with rheumatic diseases.[11] Cases were included only if sufficient information was provided to substantiate the diagnosis of PML and the rheumatic disease in question; patients were excluded if they had HIV or cancer or had undergone organ transplantation. The search revealed 50 patients with rheumatic diseases who had PML, with an overrepresentation of patients with SLE (n = 32), despite a much lower population prevalence of SLE compared with rheumatoid arthritis (n = 5). Examination of the immunosuppressive therapies prescribed to these patients within 6 months of the onset of neurologic symptoms attributed to PML revealed that low-dose (≤15 mg/d) prednisone, with or without an antimalarial agent, was the only immunosuppressive therapy in 31% of patients with SLE and 11% of patients with rheumatic diseases other than SLE. Three patients had no documented immunosuppressive therapy in the 6 months before the onset of PML.[11]

To circumvent reporting bias, a nationwide hospital discharge database representing nearly 300 million patient discharges was subsequently used to determine the relative frequency of PML in patients with rheumatic diseases.[37] Because of the reliance on diagnostic coding, rheumatic diseases were likely underreported in this sample; information on therapies was unavailable. After excluding patients with HIV or cancer and organ transplant recipients, 4 cases of PML were identified per 100,000 SLE discharges, which was 10-fold higher than the rate in rheumatoid arthritis and 20-fold higher than that of the background population.

The occurrence of PML among patients with rheumatic diseases has traditionally been attributed to the associated immunosuppressive therapy, with cyclophosphamide and other alkylating agents frequently implicated. However, these data showed that although PML is a rare occurrence in patients with rheumatic diseases, SLE was associated with a specific predisposition to PML, disproportionate to the degree of iatrogenic immunosuppression.

Lymphopenia is a manifestation of SLE, and this may be proposed as a potential explanation for an increased risk of PML in patients with SLE. However, lymphopenia is neither necessary nor sufficient for the development of PML, and a more global impairment of cell-mediated immunity, independent of immunosuppressive therapy, has not been defined in patients with SLE. A study of 20 patients with SLE investigated the prevalence of polyomaviruses in urine and plasma of patients with SLE, without any increased rates of positivity compared with controls.[38] Other studies also have failed to demonstrate aberrant handling of JCV in patients with SLE.[39,40] This emphasizes the critical role of other as yet poorly defined host factors in determining individual susceptibility to the development of PML.

Role of Specific Disease-Modifying Drugs

In PML, attributing causality to any specific immunosuppressive agent is difficult given the relative rarity of PML and the multiple confounding factors that exist in many cases. Exceptions are the monoclonal antibodies natalizumab[14] and efalizumab,[41] directed against α4 integrin and CD11a respectively, which are clearly linked to the development of PML, as emphasized in a recent stratification of therapeutic agents associated with PML.[13] The immunosuppressive therapies used to treat rheumatic disease were classified as either "Class 2, low risk of PML" (rituximab, belimumab, cyclophosphamide, azathioprine, mycophenolate, methotrexate) or "Class 3, very low risk of PML" (anti–tumor necrosis factor [TNF] therapy, tocilizumab, abatacept, ustekinumab, anakinra, tofacitinib). This discussion is limited to agents approved for treatment of rheumatic disease.

Rituximab

Rituximab is a chimeric monoclonal antibody that targets and depletes CD20-expressing cells of B-cell lineage and is approved for the treatment of rheumatoid arthritis and antineutrophil cytoplasm antibody–associated vasculitis. It is also frequently used off label for the treatment of SLE and other connective tissue disorders. Rituximab is approved for the treatment of lymphoma and has been associated with many cases of PML in that setting.[42,43] However, most of these cases are cofounded by other risk factors for PML, such as concomitant chemotherapy, bone marrow transplantation, and the underlying hematologic malignancy.

The FDA issued an alert in December 2006 following documentation of 2 fatal cases of PML in patients with SLE treated with rituximab.[36] The first case of rituximab-associated PML in the setting of rheumatoid arthritis was recorded in September 2008.[44] Additional cases were subsequently reported in a review of the literature,[45] an analysis of the FDA Adverse Event Reporting System (AERS) database through 2010[46] and an updated analysis of the AERS database through August 2012.[12] In total, 26 cases of PML were identified in patients concomitantly treated with rituximab for rheumatic disease (n = 8 for rheumatoid arthritis [RA]), although confounders were present in many cases. The discordant signal regarding the occurrence of PML among rituximab-treated patients compared with other biologic therapies is a source of concern. Nevertheless, rituximab-associated PML is a rare adverse event. It occurs in fewer than 1 in 20,000 rituximab-treated patients who have RA. Eighteen cases have occurred in the setting of other rheumatic diseases, with an unknown denominator. Clearly, ongoing vigilance is required. A better understanding of the potential mechanism responsible for the increased risk of developing PML may help in risk prediction and to guide patient selection for this agent.

Precisely how rituximab may contribute to PML pathogenesis is unclear. Humoral immunity is not protective against PML, leading to speculation that the loss of other B-cell functions, such as those of antigen-presenting cells or cytokine production, may lead to a defect in cell-mediated immunity. Houff and Berger[47] speculated that although JCV remains latent in the resting B cells in healthy individuals, B-cell–depleted patients subsequently experiencing B-cell repletion may reactivate JCV in newly developing B cells. During B-cell repletion, immature B cells undergo a series of molecular transformations, including enrichment for specific nuclear transcription factors, such as members of the NF1 family, capable of binding to the viral promoter region. These developing cells could also in some way provide a milieu, which enhances rearrangements in the virus regulatory region.[47] Again, although this theory is appealing in construct, experiments confirming or refuting this have not been reported but are urgently needed.

Belimumab

Belimumab is a monoclonal antibody directed against BlyS/BAFF, a key B-cell survival signal, approved for the treatment of SLE. The concept that B-cell directed therapies are particularly associated with the development of PML is supported by the reports of 2 cases of PML associated with use of belimumab.[48,49] A caveat is that both patients had SLE, therefore likely at some increased risk.

Anti–tumor necrosis factor therapy

In a review of the AERS database through August 2012, 4 patients with PML were identified as developing PML during anti-TNF therapy for rheumatic diseases, one of whom was concomitantly receiving cyclophosphamide, and another had significant prior cyclophosphamide exposure.[12,46] A paucity of confirmed cases in patients treated with anti-TNF therapy argues against a significant risk of PML associated with this therapy, especially considering the estimated in excess of 3 million patients with RA treated with anti-TNF agents. A note of caution is sounded by 2 additional cases of PML in patients with RA treated with adalimumab.[50,51] Ongoing vigilance is therefore necessary.

Other biologic therapies

No confirmed cases of PML in abatacept-treated patients have been published in the peer-reviewed medical literature, and no confirmed case of PML was identified in the FDA AERS database through August 2012.[12,46] However, reports of PML associated with belatacept, a closely related compound licensed for prophylaxis of transplant rejection, mandate continued vigilance for occurrence of PML in the setting of costimulatory blockade, including abatacept therapy.

There have been no cases of PML reported in association with other biologic therapies, such as tocilizumab, ustekinumab, or secukinumab to date.[12,13] However, given the rarity of PML and the relatively sparse experience with these agents, an association with PML cannot be excluded.

Synthetic (nonbiologic) immunosuppressive drugs

PML has been associated with a variety of nonbiologic immunosuppressive agents, including cyclophosphamide, azathioprine, and mycophenolate.[13,46] Although the last of these has been the subject of specific reports,[52,53] additional confounders were present in these cases (organ transplant, SLE, and/or other immunosuppressive drugs). In the FDA AERS database, all 5 confirmed cases of PML in mycophenolate-treated patients had earlier received treatment with cyclophosphamide.[46] These data suggested no clear signal of excess risk with mycophenolate above that seen with other nonbiologic immunosuppressive agents, such as cyclophosphamide or azathioprine.[13]

PREVENTIVE STRATEGIES

There are no established preventive strategies with respect to the development of PML in patients with rheumatic diseases, other than the judicious use of immunosuppressive therapies. In contrast, a useful risk stratification algorithm has been used to predict the development of PML in natalizumab-treated patients with multiple sclerosis (MS).[16] Key factors include the duration of natalizumab therapy, prior immunosuppressive therapy, and JCV seropositivity. Patients are closely monitored clinically and by serial MRI. Recent data suggest that JCV seroconversion or a rising JCV index may predate the development of PML,[54] but further confirmatory studies are required.

JCV antibody testing has not been examined in patients with rheumatic disease and is unlikely to be cost-effective in this population with a much lower incidence of PML. It would likely generate significant anxiety on behalf of patients and providers, as approximately half of all patients will test positive, only a tiny minority of whom will subsequently develop PML. The reliability of testing is also limited by the occurrence of false-negative tests.[55] This might lead to avoidance or underutilization of effective therapies for the underlying rheumatic disease.

MANAGEMENT
Restore Immune Function

The critical element for survival in PML is reversal of the immunosuppressive state if possible. In non-HIV–infected patients, such as those with rheumatic disease, prompt diagnosis followed by reducing or eliminating immunosuppression is prudent and may improve outcomes. This is particularly relevant, as many patients are initially misdiagnosed with a flare or new onset of a neuroinflammatory manifestation of their underlying autoimmune disease and consequently exposed to increased immunosuppression.[11,46] Increased awareness of this rare but serious complication should reduce the frequency of this error in management.

Plasmapheresis may improve outcomes by enhancing drug clearance in natalizumab-treated patients with MS who develop PML[56]; however, this has not been established for other biologic therapies. It is not likely that plasmapheresis would be of value in patients who develop PML following rituximab therapy given the long interval that typically exists between last rituximab infusion and the development of PML (median 5 months).[12,46]

Rule Out Human Immunodeficiency Virus

All patients diagnosed with PML should be screened for HIV, as it represents a treatable underlying cause for the development of PML. Institution of HAART can improve outcomes and reduce mortality in HIV-infected patients with PML.[56]

Drug Therapy for Progressive Multifocal Leukoencephalopathy

Mirtazapine and mefloquine are frequently prescribed but are unproven.[56,57] The use of antiviral agents, such as cytarabine, cidofovir, or others, is unproven and must be weighed individually.[56] The recent reports of use of immune-stimulant strategies involving interleukin (IL)-2 and IL-7 are of interest but remain experimental.[58–60] Potential future strategies include gene editing.[61,62]

SUMMARY

PML has been reported in association with a variety of rheumatic diseases, although a predisposition in patients with SLE has become apparent. Synthetic and biologic immunosuppressive therapies have also been implicated, but PML may also occur in the setting of minimal iatrogenic immunosuppression. The rarity of PML indicates that in addition to disease-related and treatment-related immunosuppression, as yet ill-defined host factors play a key role in disease susceptibility. Until greater clarity can be achieved, all patients with systemic rheumatic diseases should be considered at risk for PML, regardless of the nature or intensity of their immunosuppressive therapy. PML should be considered in patients with unexplained subacute progressive focal and diffuse neurologic deficits, especially if their clinical or radiologic status worsens in the face of increased intensity of immunosuppressive therapy. In this context, differentiating PML from neurologic syndromes related to the underlying rheumatic disease is critical, particularly given the markedly different approaches to management. Ongoing vigilance for and reporting of cases of PML in patients with rheumatic disease treated with synthetic or biologic therapies are essential to enhance the understanding of the associated risk. There are no reliable preventive strategies for PML in the setting of rheumatic disease other than the judicious use of immunosuppressive therapies. There is no established therapeutic strategy in patients with rheumatic disease who develop PML, other than restoration of immune function through withdrawal of immunosuppressive therapy.

REFERENCES

1. Tan CS, Koralnik IJ. Progressive multifocal leukoencephalopathy and other disorders caused by JC virus: clinical features and pathogenesis. Lancet Neurol 2010; 9(4):425–37.

2. Johne R, Buck CB, Allander T, et al. Taxonomical developments in the family Polyomaviridae. Arch Virol 2011;156(9):1627–34.

3. Wollebo HS, White MK, Gordon J, et al. Persistence and pathogenesis of the neurotropic polyomavirus JC. Ann Neurol 2015;77(4):560–70.

4. Brew BJ, Davies NWS, Cinque P, et al. Progressive multifocal leukoencephalopathy and other forms of JC virus disease. Nat Rev Neurol 2010;6(12):667–79.

5. White MK, Khalili K. Pathogenesis of progressive multifocal leukoencephalopathy–revisited. J Infect Dis 2011;203(5):578–86.

6. Bayliss J, Karasoulos T, Bowden S, et al. Immunosuppression increases latent infection of brain by JC polyomavirus. Pathology 2011;43(4):362–7.

7. Bayliss J, Karasoulos T, McLean CA. Immunosuppression increases JC polyoma virus large T antigen DNA load in the brains of patients without progressive multifocal leukoencephalopathy. J Infect Dis 2013;207(1):133–6.

8. Berger JR, Khalili K. The pathogenesis of progressive multifocal leukoencephalopathy. Discov Med 2011;12(67):495–503.

9. Gheuens S, Pierone G, Peeters P, et al. Progressive multifocal leukoencephalopathy in individuals with minimal or occult immunosuppression. J Neurol Neurosurg Psychiatry 2010;81(3):247–54.

10. Tan IL, Koralnik IJ, Rumbaugh JA, et al. Progressive multifocal leukoencephalopathy in a patient without immunodeficiency. Neurology 2011;77(3):297–9.

11. Calabrese LH, Molloy ES, Huang D, et al. Progressive multifocal leukoencephalopathy in rheumatic diseases: evolving clinical and pathologic patterns of disease. Arthritis Rheum 2007;56(7):2116–28.

12. Molloy ES, Calabrese LH. Progressive multifocal leukoencephalopathy associated with biologic therapy in rheumatic diseases: strengthening association with rituximab. Arthritis Rheumatol 2014;66:S369.

13. Calabrese LH, Molloy E, Berger J. Sorting out the risks in progressive multifocal leukoencephalopathy. Nat Rev Rheumatol 2015;11(2):119–23.

14. Major EO. Progressive multifocal leukoencephalopathy in patients on immunomodulatory therapies. Annu Rev Med 2010;61:35–47.

15. Durali D, de Goër de Herve MG, Gasnault J, et al. B cells and progressive multifocal leukoencephalopathy: search for the missing link. Front Immunol 2015;6:241.

16. Gorelik L, Lerner M, Bixler S, et al. Anti-JC virus antibodies: implications for PML risk stratification. Ann Neurol 2010;68(3):295–303.

17. Clifford DB. Neurological immune reconstitution inflammatory response: riding the tide of immune recovery. Curr Opin Neurol 2015;28(3):295–301.

18. Berger JR. The basis for modeling progressive multifocal leukoencephalopathy pathogenesis. Curr Opin Neurol 2011;24(3):262–7.

19. Lima MA, Drislane FW, Koralnik IJ. Seizures and their outcome in progressive multifocal leukoencephalopathy. Neurology 2006;66(2):262–4.

20. Küker W, Mader I, Nägele T, et al. Progressive multifocal leukoencephalopathy: value of diffusion-weighted and contrast-enhanced magnetic resonance imaging for diagnosis and treatment control. Eur J Neurol 2006;13(8):819–26.

21. Lima MA, Hanto DW, Curry MP, et al. Atypical radiological presentation of progressive multifocal leukoencephalopathy following liver transplantation. J Neurovirol 2005;11(1):46–50.

22. Rosas MJ, Simões-Ribeiro F, An SF, et al. Progressive multifocal leukoencephalopathy: unusual MRI findings and prolonged survival in a pregnant woman. Neurology 1999;52(3):657–9.

23. Post MJ, Yiannoutsos C, Simpson D, et al. Progressive multifocal leukoencephalopathy in AIDS: are there any MR findings useful to patient management and predictive of patient survival? AIDS Clinical Trials Group, 243 Team. AJNR Am J Neuroradiol 1999;20(10):1896–906.

24. Huang D, Cossoy M, Li M, et al. Inflammatory progressive multifocal leukoencephalopathy in human immunodeficiency virus-negative patients. Ann Neurol 2007;62(1):34–9.

25. Cinque P, Vago L, Dahl H, et al. Polymerase chain reaction on cerebrospinal fluid for diagnosis of virus-associated opportunistic diseases of the central nervous system in HIV-infected patients. AIDS 1996;10(9):951–8.

26. Di Giambenedetto S, Vago G, Pompucci A, et al. Fatal inflammatory AIDS-associated PML with high CD4 counts on HAART: a new clinical entity? Neurology 2004;63(12):2452–3.

27. Martinez JV, Mazziotti JV, Efron ED, et al. Immune reconstitution inflammatory syndrome associated with PML in AIDS: a treatable disorder. Neurology 2006;67(9): 1692–4.

28. Langer-Gould A, Atlas SW, Green AJ, et al. Progressive multifocal leukoencephalopathy in a patient treated with natalizumab. N Engl J Med 2005;353(4):375–81.

29. Zivanovic M, Savšek L, Poljak M, et al. Possible pitfalls in the diagnostic of progressive multifocal leukoencephalopathy. Clin Neuropathol 2016;35(2):66–71.

30. Calabrese LH, Molloy ES, Taege AJ. Rheumatologists knowledge, attitudes and concerns regarding progressive multifocal leukoencephalopathy. Arthritis Rheum 2009;60(S10):130.

31. Nived O, Bengtsson AA, Jönsen A, et al. Progressive multifocal leukoencephalopathy—the importance of early diagnosis illustrated in four cases. Lupus 2008;17(11):1036–41.

32. Greenan TJ, Grossman RI, Goldberg HI. Cerebral vasculitis: MR imaging and angiographic correlation. Radiology 1992;182(1):65–72.

33. Harris KG, Tran DD, Sickels WJ, et al. Diagnosing intracranial vasculitis: the roles of MR and angiography. AJNR Am J Neuroradiol 1994;15(2):317–30.

34. Finelli PF, Onyiuke HC, Uphoff DF. Idiopathic granulomatous angiitis of the CNS manifesting as diffuse white matter disease. Neurology 1997;49(6):1696–9.

35. Sibbitt WL, Brooks WM, Kornfeld M, et al. Magnetic resonance imaging and brain histopathology in neuropsychiatric systemic lupus erythematosus. Semin Arthritis Rheum 2010;40(1):32–52.

36. Rituxan warning. FDA Consum 2007;41(2):3.

37. Molloy ES, Calabrese LH. Progressive multifocal leukoencephalopathy: a national estimate of frequency in systemic lupus erythematosus and other rheumatic diseases. Arthritis Rheum 2009;60(12):3761–5.

38. Sundsfjord A, Osei A, Rosenqvist H, et al. BK and JC viruses in patients with systemic lupus erythematosus: prevalent and persistent BK viruria, sequence stability of the viral regulatory regions, and nondetectable viremia. J Infect Dis 1999; 180(1):1–9.

39. Iacobaeus E, Hopia L, Khademi M, et al. Analysis of JC virus DNA in NPSLE patients treated with different immunomodulatory agents. Lupus 2013;22(3):307–11.

40. Bendiksen S, Rekvig OP, Van Ghelue M, et al. VP1 DNA sequences of JC and BK viruses detected in urine of systemic lupus erythematosus patients reveal no differences from strains expressed in normal individuals. J Gen Virol 2000;81(Pt 11): 2625–33.

41. Molloy ES, Calabrese LH. Therapy: targeted but not trouble-free: efalizumab and PML. Nat Rev Rheumatol 2009;5(8):418–9.

42. Carson KR, Evens AM, Richey EA, et al. Progressive multifocal leukoencephalopathy after rituximab therapy in HIV-negative patients: a report of 57 cases from the Research on Adverse Drug Events and Reports project. Blood 2009; 113(20):4834–40.

43. Tuccori M, Focosi D, Blandizzi C, et al. Inclusion of rituximab in treatment protocols for non-Hodgkin's lymphomas and risk for progressive multifocal leukoencephalopathy. Oncologist 2010;15(11):1214–9.

44. Fleischmann RM. Progressive multifocal leukoencephalopathy following rituximab treatment in a patient with rheumatoid arthritis. Arthritis Rheum 2009; 60(11):3225–8.

45. Clifford DB, Ances B, Costello C, et al. Rituximab-associated progressive multifocal leukoencephalopathy in rheumatoid arthritis. Arch Neurol 2011;68(9): 1156–64.

46. Molloy ES, Calabrese LH. Progressive multifocal leukoencephalopathy associated with immunosuppressive therapy in rheumatic diseases: evolving role of biologic therapies. Arthritis Rheum 2012;64(9):3043–51.

47. Houff SA, Berger JR. The bone marrow, B cells, and JC virus. J Neurovirol 2008; 14(5):341–3.

48. Fredericks CA, Kvam KA, Bear J, et al. A case of progressive multifocal leukoencephalopathy in a lupus patient treated with belimumab. Lupus 2014;23(7):711–3.

49. Leblanc-Trudeau C, Masetto A, Bocti C. Progressive multifocal leukoencephalopathy associated with belimumab in a patient with systemic lupus erythematosus. J Rheumatol 2015;42(3):551–2.

50. Ray M, Curtis JR, Baddley JW. A case report of progressive multifocal leucoencephalopathy (PML) associated with adalimumab. Ann Rheum Dis 2014;73(7): 1429–30.

51. Babi MA, Pendlebury W, Braff S, et al. JC virus PCR detection is not infallible: a fulminant case of progressive multifocal leukoencephalopathy with false-negative cerebrospinal fluid studies despite progressive clinical course and radiological findings. Case Rep Neurol Med 2015;2015:643216.

52. Communication About an Ongoing Safety Review of CellCept (mycophenolate mofetil) and Myfortic (mycophenolic acid). U.S Food and Drug Administration. MedWatch. The FDA Safety Information and Adverse Event Reporting Program. 2009. Available at: http://www.fda.gov/Drugs/DrugSafety/PostmarketDrugSafetyInformationforPati entsandProviders/DrugSafetyInformationforHeathcareProfessionals/ucm072438.htm. Accessed June 28, 2011.

53. Neff RT, Hurst FP, Falta EM, et al. Progressive multifocal leukoencephalopathy and use of mycophenolate mofetil after kidney transplantation. Transplantation 2008;86(10):1474–8.

54. Plavina T, Berman M, Njenga M, et al. Multi-site analytical validation of an assay to detect anti-JCV antibodies in human serum and plasma. J Clin Virol 2012; 53(1):65–71.

55. Berger JR, Houff SA, Gurwell J, et al. JC virus antibody status underestimates infection rates. Ann Neurol 2013;74(1):84–90.

56. Clifford DB. Progressive multifocal leukoencephalopathy therapy. J Neurovirol 2015;21(6):632–6.

57. Clifford DB, Nath A, Cinque P, et al. A study of mefloquine treatment for progressive multifocal leukoencephalopathy: results and exploration of predictors of PML outcomes. J Neurovirol 2013;19(4):351–8.

58. Dubey D, Zhang Y, Graves D, et al. Use of interleukin-2 for management of natalizumab-associated progressive multifocal leukoencephalopathy: case report and review of literature. Ther Adv Neurol Disord 2016;9(3):211–5.

59. Sospedra M, Schippling S, Yousef S, et al. Treating progressive multifocal leukoencephalopathy with interleukin 7 and vaccination with JC virus capsid protein VP1. Clin Infect Dis 2014;59(11):1588–92.

60. Miskin DP, Chalkias SG, Dang X, et al. Interleukin-7 treatment of PML in a patient with idiopathic lymphocytopenia. Neurol Neuroimmunol Neuroinflamm 2016;3(2): e213.

61. Wollebo HS, Bellizzi A, Kaminski R, et al. CRISPR/Cas9 system as an agent for eliminating polyomavirus JC infection. PLoS One 2015;10(9):e0136046.

62. White MK, Kaminski R, Wollebo H, et al. Gene editing for treatment of neurological infections. Neurotherapeutics 2016;13(3):547–54.

Incidence and Prevention of Herpes Zoster Reactivation in Patients with Autoimmune Diseases

Eliza F. Chakravarty, MD, MS

KEYWORDS

- Herpes zoster • Varicella zoster virus • Reactivation • Autoimmune disease
- Vaccine • Rheumatoid arthritis • Systemic lupus erythematosus
- Immunosuppression

KEY POINTS

- 98% of the adult population in the United States has serologic evidence of primary varicella zoster virus infection, and presumably host latent virus in the dorsal ganglia.
- Latent VZV virus is kept in check by cell mediated immunity, which wanes slowly over time.
- Individuals with lupus and rheumatoid arthritis have higher incidence of herpes zoster compared to age matched controls.
- Dissecting the role of underlying immune dysregulation of rheumatic diseases from the use of immunosuppressive medications in the risk of herpes zoster is difficult.
- A live-attenuated virus vaccine is currently available to reduce the incidence and severity of herpes zoster in adults >50 years old.
- Although theoretical risks of developing clinical zoster from the vaccine-strain of VZV remain, current studies are underway to determine the safety and efficacy of zoster vaccination in the high risk of population.

Herpes zoster (HZ), also called zoster and shingles, is caused by reactivation of latent varicella zoster virus (VZV) that usually occurs decades following initial exposure. Before 1995, most people were infected as children and developed the clinical syndrome of chicken pox, although some individuals have anti-VZV antibodies without recall of clinically evident disease. In 1995, a live-attenuated vaccine against VZV (Varivax, Merck) was introduced in the United States and became part of the routine

Conflicts of Interest: None.
Funding Sources: Oklahoma Center for the Advancement of Science and Technology, HR12-064.
Arthritis and Clinical Immunology, Oklahoma Medical Research Foundation, 825 Northeast 13th Street, Oklahoma City, OK 73104, USA
E-mail address: chakravartye@omrf.org

Rheum Dis Clin N Am 43 (2017) 111–121
http://dx.doi.org/10.1016/j.rdc.2016.09.010

childhood vaccine schedule, with the first dose administered at 13 to 15 months of age. Approximately 98% of the adult population in the United States has serologic evidence of primary infection with varicella[1] and is therefore at risk for the later development of zoster. Although the vaccine is approximately 85% effective, many children develop clinical or subclinical infection with wild-type virus, and are still at risk for later HZ. Although rare, localized or disseminated OKA (vaccine-strain) varicella, and even later HZ can develop in Varivax-vaccinated children.[2] Clinically, zoster typically presents as a unilateral vesicular rash limited to 1 or 2 dermatomes, usually in the thoracic, cervical, and ophthalmologic regions. The rash usually lasts 7 to 10 days, during which the virus may be transmissible through airborne particles. Complications of zoster include postherpetic neuralgia, bacterial superinfection, and disseminated zoster with meningoencephalitis. The incidence of zoster increases with age, presumably because cell-mediated immunity (CMI) wanes with advancing age. Studies of VZV CMI in unvaccinated individuals estimate an approximate 2.7% to 3.9% decrease with each year of age after 60 years, whereas VZV-specific antibody levels remain essentially unchanged.[3] The age-adjusted incidence of zoster in the general population in the United States is estimated to be 3.6 to 4.4 per 1000 person-years,[4,5] with rates highest among elderly individuals, reaching 11.0 per 1000 person-years in women more than 65 years of age.[5] Women seem to be more susceptible to HZ reactivation than men, with an approximate 25% to 30% higher incidence among women at all ages.[3–5] Studies have suggested that the sex difference in HZ incidence may be explained by a lower frequency of VZV-specific memory T cells in women.[6]

The Centers for Disease Control and Prevention (CDC) published guidelines for the use of the US Food and Drug Administration (FDA)–approved live-attenuated HZ vaccine (Zostavax, Merck), which is the identical OKA/Merck strain of the Varivax vaccine, but has 14 times the potency to account for the immunosenescence of advancing age and prior exposure to VZV.[1] This document outlines recommendations as well as relative contraindications for the use of the zoster vaccine in adults in the United States, particularly for immunocompromised individuals. Note that these recommendations are based on theoretic concerns, and not based on human data of adverse events of zoster vaccine administration in immunocompromised persons. Guidelines suggest that the vaccine may not be contraindicated for people taking low-dose corticosteroids (<20 mg prednisone daily equivalent), methotrexate ($\leq$0.4 mg/kg/wk), azathioprine ($\leq$3.0 mg/kg/d), or 6-mercaptopurine ($\leq$1.5 mg/kg/d). The decision to vaccinate individuals who are concurrently receiving biologic therapies, particularly tumor necrosis factor inhibitors (TNFi), should be made on an individual basis, but, if possible, the vaccine should be given 4 weeks before institution of biologic therapy. There is no mention of vaccinating individuals who are currently receiving mycophenolate mofetil, which is one of the most commonly used medications for moderate-to-severe systemic lupus erythematosus (SLE).[1]

Unlike influenza, the antibody response to varicella virus does not protect against reactivation of latent virus. It is presumed that the immunoglobulin (Ig) G antibody response serves to protect the host from reexposure of exogenous virus at sites of inoculation after contact with infected individuals.[7] Therefore, the presence of VZV-specific IgG antibodies correlates with past exposure to varicella or effective vaccination, and protects against primary infection.[8] Seroconversion following vaccination is associated with protection from primary vaccination, and loss of detectable antibodies places the individual at risk for breakthrough infection.[8]

In contrast, it seems that intact VZV-specific T cell–mediated immunity is critical to protection from reactivation of latent varicella infection of sensory ganglia following initial infection. In healthy elderly adults, the incidence of HZ reactivation increases with age despite fairly consistent anti-VZV antibody titers. Individuals with T-cell immunodeficiencies, either congenital, acquired immunodeficiency syndrome related, or via immunosuppressive medications, are at increased risk for inability to resolve acute infection, development of life-threatening infection, or frequent episodes of viral reactivation. However, individuals with B-cell immunodeficiency syndromes do not seem to have increased susceptibility to infection or reactivation.[7] At present, the most common assay for VZV-specific cell-mediated immunity in both clinical trials and observational studies is the interferon gamma (IFNγ)–secreting enzyme linked immunosorbent SPOT (ELISPOT) assay, a modification of the enzyme-linked immunosorbent assay that enumerates cytokine production by single cells following stimulation.[9] In an immunologic substudy of the randomized, placebo-controlled Shingles Prevention Study, all 1395 participants had detectable VZV IgG antibodies at baseline, whereas 18.5% had undetectable IFNγ ELISPOT assays. The decline in VZV-specific IFNγ ELISPOT response was approximately 3.9% per increased year of age.[3]

SYSTEMIC LUPUS ERYTHEMATOSUS

Several studies have shown that zoster is more common, and can present with more severe manifestations, among immunocompromised patients, including those with SLE and rheumatoid arthritis (RA) with various degrees of immunosuppressive medications.[10–21] Evidence suggests that the incidence of zoster may be increased in these autoimmune diseases even in the absence of immunosuppressive medications.[11,17] This increase is possibly caused by an inherent deficiency in cell-mediated or other immunity associated with the disease process. However, distinctions between susceptibility from immunosuppressive medications and susceptibility caused by intrinsic immunologic defects inherent in autoimmune diseases remain elusive.

The autoimmune disease with the most compelling epidemiologic evidence of increased risk of HZ is SLE. Most estimates of the incidence of HZ in SLE have been derived from retrospective single-center studies. Studies have estimated the annual incidence of zoster to range from 6.4/1000 person-years to 32.5/1000 in patients with SLE.[11,16,21] This is nearly 2-fold to 10-fold more than the estimated rate of zoster in the general population of 3.4/1000 person-years to 4.4/1000 person-years. In a large study of governmentally and commercially insured adults, the incidence rate of HZ among people with SLE ranged from 15.2 to 24.6 cases per 1000 person-years, with increased rates distributed across all age groups. This rate is significantly higher than is found for healthy individuals aged 61 to 70 years (8.5/1000 person-years) and aged 71 years and older (10.6/1000 person-years); individuals for whom the shingles vaccine is indicated.[22] Furthermore, age-adjusted and gender-adjusted standardized incidence rates for HZ in SLE approach 20/1000 person-years; nearly 4-fold higher than healthy individuals (5.5/1000 person-years) or those with diabetes mellitus (7.5/1000 person-years).[21] In juvenile-onset SLE, estimates approach 58.7/1000 person-years.[23]

Studies are mixed regarding relative roles of SLE disease activity and immunosuppressive medications in increasing risk of HZ. Some studies have found that certain immunosuppressive medications, such as glucocorticoids, azathioprine, and cyclophosphamide, increase the risk of HZ, as would be expected based on the degree of immunosuppression caused by these agents. Among patients with SLE, use of prednisone (hazard ratio [HR], 2.29; 95% confidence interval [CI], 1.24–4.23) and mycophenolate mofetil (HR, 5.0; 95% CI, 1.4–17.6) within the past 6 months placed patients at higher risk for developing HZ. Another case-control study of HZ in SLE performed in a nationwide sample from Taiwan found that use of any immunomodulatory or immunosuppressant medication, including hydroxychloroquine, increased the risk of HZ in a dose-dependent manner.[24] Studies are generally mixed, with some showing HZ incidence increasing with immunosuppression, whereas others found a high rate of HZ among patients with SLE with quiescent disease on little to no immunosuppression.[12,15,21,25] In another study of large administrative claims data, the crude incidence of HZ among all patients with SLE was estimated to be 15.2/1000 person-years compared with 4.8/1000 person-years in the general population.[26] Although the use of immunosuppressant therapy among patients with SLE increased the incidence of HZ further, even those patients with SLE not receiving immunosuppressants had increased HZ compared with the general population (12.2/1000 person-years),[26] suggesting that immunosuppressants play a smaller role in the increased risk of HZ imposed by SLE.

Very few studies have evaluated the role of VZV-specific immunity in SLE in relation to risk of HZ reactivation. One study of 24 Korean patients with SLE, all anti-VZV IgG positive, found statistically significantly lower VZV-specific IFNγ-releasing CD4 cells (0.043% ± 0.009%) than in 12 healthy subjects (0.126% ± 0.025%; $P = .007$).[11] Cell-mediated responses to cytomegalovirus among patients with SLE were higher, suggesting that the lower response to VZV may be more specific than simply a general reduction in surveillance against viral infections. However, rates of HZ in this cohort were not reported.

One group published the results of a pilot study of CMI response to the live-attenuated HZ vaccine (Zostavax) in 10 female patients with SLE with quiescent disease and on minimal immunosuppressant medications (following CDC guidelines) compared with responses in healthy women.[27] Although not designed for statistical power, the study found that patients with SLE mounted a demonstrable, but lower-magnitude, VZV-specific response than healthy women at 2, 6, and 12 weeks after vaccination. The proportion of subjects in each group with a greater than 50% increase in VZV-specific CMI compared with baseline was similar at all time points following vaccination, with no VZV-related adverse events or flares of underlying SLE. Patients with SLE seemed to have a blunted CMI response to VZV exposure, and this may, in part, contribute to the increased rates of HZ seen in this population. However, reasons for the blunted response have yet to be explored.

Rheumatoid Arthritis

RA is an autoimmune disease with a much higher prevalence than SLE in the population, with a later mean age of onset and a lower female/male ratio. Newer biologic and small-molecule therapies that are now in widespread use because of their efficacy in controlling signs and symptoms and slowing the progression of damage among patients with RA have brought with them increasing concerns about susceptibility to infections, including HZ.

Cumulative evidence from many studies has indicated that patients with RA carry a 1.5-fold to 2-fold increased risk of HZ compared with age-matched healthy adults, and these results have been consistent over several decades of follow-up as therapeutic regimens and options have changed for these patients. As expected, increasing age, female sex, glucocorticoid use, and poor functional status were associated with increased risk.[13,26,28] The incidence of HZ in patients with RA who were not receiving immune-suppressant therapy was still increased compared with the general population (9.6/1000 person-years compared with 4.8/1000 person-years) in a large administrative claims study that followed individuals from 2005 to 2009.[26] The risk was increased for patients with RA receiving immunosuppressive therapy (not analyzed by therapeutic agent or class) to 14.3/1000 person-years, resulting in an overall incidence of HZ among patients with RA of 12.2/1000 person-years.[26]

Similarly, in the study by Yun and colleagues[22] comparing HZ rates by age group, patients with RA aged 40 years and older reached the incidence threshold of 8.5/1000 person-years (incidence of HZ for healthy adults aged $\geq$61 years) for whom HZ vaccination is indicated.

With the advent and widespread use of TNFi at the turn of the century came increased concerns for infection risk given an increased level of immunosuppression greater than what would be expected by traditional disease-modifying antirheumatic drugs (DMARDs), including methotrexate, leflunomide, sulfasalazine, and hydroxylchloroquine. An epidemiologic study of HZ in patients with RA conducted early in the TNFi era found that prednisone, leflunomide, and azathioprine use increased HZ risk, but not any of the available TNFi (etanercept, infliximab, and adalimumab).[13] In the Yun and colleagues[22] study across several autoimmune diseases, a multivariate analysis to identify risk factors for HZ among patients with RA found a slight increase (HR, 1.18; 95% CI, 1.04–1.34) with the use of biologic medications as a class, which was remarkably lower than any use of glucocorticoids (HR 1.63, 95% CI 1.44–1.85 for 5 mg daily; and HR 2.15, 95% CI 1.87–2.48 for $\geq$5 mg prednisone daily).[21] This study followed health care recipients between the years 2007 and 2010, when non-TNFi biologics were still used sparingly. A similar study by the same group evaluated incidence of HZ among Medicare recipients with RA from 2006 to 2011 for associations with different RA biologic therapies.[29] Following that study, an observational longitudinal study of more than 28,000 US patients with RA enrolled in the Corrona Registry between 2001 and 2013 compared incidence of HZ by biologic therapy (TNFi; non-TNFi, including rituximab, abatacept, tocilizumab, and anakinra; compared with traditional DMARDs).[28] The overall incidence of HZ was 7.7/1000 person-years. In multivariable analyses, increasing age, prednisone use, and physical function were independently associated with increased incidence of HZ, whereas no statistically significant differences were identified between the treatment categories. These associations remained after adjustment for other medical comorbidities and for propensity scores for the use of the different RA therapies.[28] In contrast with reassuring data from the United States, recent data for the risk of HZ in RA worldwide has suggested an increased risk associated with TNFi use, with HRs for TNFi exposure ranging from 1.61 to 2.33 compared with patients taking traditional DMARDs.[30–32]

A more recent study evaluated health plan administrative data from 2010 to 2014 to compare risks of HZ among patients with RA with a specific focus on newer biologic and small-molecule therapies.[33] There was no comparator group of patients with RA who were not taking any DMARD therapy or who were only receiving traditional, prebiologic DMARDs. The largest exposure was to TNFi (combined) with 27,122 person-years of observation. Multivariable analysis, adjusting for age, sex, glucocorticoid use, hospitalizations, and history of zoster vaccination, found that only tofacitinib (a small-molecule janus kinase [JAK]-3/JAK-1 inhibitor) had an increased risk of HZ, with an HR of 1.40 (95% CI, 1.09–1.81) compared with all other biologic agents, including TNFi, abatacept, rituximab, and tocilizumab,[33] suggesting a possible mechanism specific to JAK inhibition that contributes to the increased risk compared with RA or with generalized immunosuppression with other typical RA therapies. The specific concern of HZ with tofacitinib had been raised earlier, after analysis of the international tofacitinib RA development program identified an incidence rate of 44/1000 person-years among patients receiving tofacitinib compared with 28/1000 person-years for adalimumab, and 15/1000 person-years for those in the placebo arm.[34] Although rates were higher with tofacitinib use, the incidence of HZ was high in all arms of this analysis of clinical trial and long-term extension studies. However, similar to all studies of HZ in autoimmune diseases, cases of disseminated disease or internal organ involvement were rare. It is postulated that inhibition of type I and type II IFN signaling through the JAK-1 receptor may underlie this potential tofacitinib-mediated susceptibility to HZ; however, specific mechanisms of increased VZV reactivation with this or other immunosuppressive medications have yet to be completely understood.

HERPES ZOSTER VACCINATION

Irrespective of the exact mechanisms underlying increased incidence of HZ in SLE and patients with RA caused by disease or immunosuppressive therapy, a live-attenuated vaccine is now commercially available that may help to reduce the burden of HZ in these populations. However, the only HZ vaccine currently available is the live-attenuated Zostavax vaccine, consisting of the OKA/Merck strain of VZV that is similarly in wide use to protect children starting at 12 to 15 months against the primary infection called chicken pox. Because the vaccine is not recombinant but a live-attenuated virus, there is a theoretic risk of an immunocompromised subject developing clinical infection from the vaccine. Most live-attenuated vaccines are considered contraindicated for immunocompromised persons, although the degree of immunosuppression to render an individual susceptible has not been described. For this reason, most rheumatologists counsel patients with RA or SLE, particularly those on moderate to high daily doses of glucocorticoids or other immunosuppressive agents, against vaccination with live-virus vaccines: bacille Calmette-Guérin for tuberculosis; oral polio vaccine; and vaccines against measles, rotavirus, varicella zoster, and yellow fever. For adults in the United States, avoiding live-attenuated virus vaccines is not particularly troubling, because immunocompromised adults are cautioned against and can easily avoid endemic areas for most of these pathogens. However, VZV is different because the exposure is endogenous and risks of HZ are known to be increased in SLE and RA populations.

Ideally, vaccination against HZ should proceed before initiation of high-dose glucocorticoids or other immunosuppressant therapies, and therapy should be delayed for at least 14 days after vaccination. Otherwise, it has been recommended that individuals be vaccinated after cessation of biologic or other immunosuppressive medications for 4 to 6 weeks, followed by reinstitution of chronic RA or SLE therapy 14 days later. However, in many circumstances this is not feasible, and it has the risk of worsening the underlying autoimmune disease. Initial onset or flares of these disease can be profound and occasionally life or organ threatening, necessitating emergent immunosuppressant treatment to ameliorate symptoms and discomfort and attempt to induce remission or retard organ dysfunction. In such cases, delaying vaccination may have negative consequences for 2 reasons: active disease remains undertreated or untreated during the vaccination period; and it is not clear how much the efficacy of any vaccine will be diminished by uncontrolled, active autoimmune or inflammatory disease. Similarly, a drug holiday primarily for the purpose of vaccination may be ill advised because it may allow disease reactivation or a flare in a new organ system that may not have occurred if maintenance therapy was not disrupted. Such a flare may lead to further requirements of higher immunosuppression and place the patient at additional risk. Therefore, until recombinant or subunit HZ vaccines are available, it is critical to better understand the degree of risk imposed by Zostavax vaccination in patients with SLE and RA on chronic, maintenance immunosuppressive therapy, and how that risk compares with the risk of developing HZ in the absence of vaccination.

At present, rates of HZ vaccination among people with RA or SLE remain extremely low, partly because of concerns about the risk of developing infection, and also because the vaccine is currently not FDA approved for people less than 50 years old. However, even among patients aged 60 years and older (for whom the vaccine is not only FDA approved but CDC recommended) the rate is extremely low: less than 5% of patients with RA,[29] and less than 13% for SLE.[18]

Clinical data on effectiveness or safety of Zostavax in these populations are sparse. The Zostavax vaccine was licensed in the United States based on a large double-blind randomized, placebo-controlled clinical trial of more than 38,000 adults aged 60 years or older.[35] This study showed a 51% reduction in the incidence of HZ among vaccinated participants, as well as a 66% reduction in postherpetic neuralgia. No episodes of vaccine-induced HZ infection occurred. Similar studies have not been performed in individuals with RA or SLE for several reasons: theoretic concerns and relative contraindication of use of live-virus vaccine preparations, and the large sample size and long follow-up required to show a reduction in incidence of HZ. However, by using administrative claims data on large groups of people, estimates of safety and reduction of HZ among vaccinated individuals may be suggested. A retrospective cohort study of more than 460,000 Medicare beneficiaries with a diagnosis of RA or other inflammatory diseases was performed to better understand the effects of Zostavax vaccination.[36] All subjects were at least 60 years old and were thus eligible to receive the vaccine. The study identified 18,683 participants who received the HZ vaccine (4.0% of the study population), and 633 subjects who were receiving biologic therapies (551 on TNFi) at the time of vaccination. None of the biologic-exposed participants developed HZ within 42 days of vaccination (the presumed vulnerable window for developing vaccine-strain clinical infection). When comparing incidence of HZ among individuals never vaccinated or before vaccination with the person-years of observation after vaccination, Zostavax vaccination reduced the incidence of HZ by approximately 40% (HR for vaccination 0.61; 95% CI, 0.52–0.71). This result is less than the 50% seen in the Shingles Prevention Study, but nonetheless showed a reasonable response to the vaccine in individuals with RA or other inflammatory diseases.[36]

A separate retrospective cohort study specifically evaluated the safety of Zostavax among current or remote users of immunosuppressive therapies for several autoimmune or inflammatory diseases using managed care organizations affiliated with the Vaccine Safety Datalink.[37] Again, vaccinated individuals were all aged 50 years and older. The study identified 14,554 vaccinated individuals, 4826 of whom were currently receiving immunosuppressant therapy compared with 9728 who had received immunosuppressant therapy within the past year, but not within 30 days of HZ vaccination. There were no cases of disseminated zoster among vaccinated individuals within 42 days of vaccination. A total of 42 cases of HZ were reported within 42 days of vaccination among the 14,000 individuals. Rates of HZ in the 42 days following vaccination were similar to rates observed in RA and other autoimmune diseases overall, although the incidence was higher in those currently receiving immunosuppressive therapy compared with remote users, which may be more of a reflection of the natural history of HZ in people with autoimmune diseases rather than a short-term effect of vaccination.[37]

A small pilot study of Zostavax administered to individuals 50 years of age and older with inflammatory bowel disease, similar in design to the study of Zostavax in SLE, again found a diminished, but measurable, immunogenic response to vaccination without evidence of HZ-related adverse events.[38] Again, the small sample size greatly limits the ability to generalize, but results are similar to the retrospective analyses of claims data that found a lower, but still meaningful, reduction in HZ incidence following vaccination in patients with RA without significant risks of live-vaccine–related adverse events.[36] In order to confirm these findings, a multicenter randomized double-blind study of Zostavax or placebo in patients with RA greater than 50 years old currently receiving TNFi is currently enrolling.[39] Goals of this study are to evaluate VZV-specific T-cell immunogenicity at 6 weeks, and to compare rates of HZ for 2 years following vaccination.

Alternatives to Live-Virus Vaccines

Given the current dilemma of using a live-attenuated vaccine preparation in immunocompromised individuals who have a demonstrable higher risk of infection, the search for vaccine alternatives has a high priority. Two alternative vaccine strategies, heat-inactivated vaccine or subunit vaccine, have been explored but are not currently commercially available. A heat-inactivated version of the OKA/Merck Varivax vaccine (V212) has been developed specifically to avoid risks of live-attenuated virus administration to immunocompromised individuals. Phase III studies of this vaccine are currently underway in adults with underlying malignancies; however, recognized limitations of this vaccine include a requirement of 4 doses to achieve an immune response compared with the response seen with Zostavax in immunocompetent people.[40] GlaxoSmithKline recently published results of a phase III randomized, placebo-controlled, double-blind study of its adjuvanted recombinant subunit HZ vaccine in 15,411 immunocompetent individuals aged 50 years and older.[41] This vaccine is composed of the VZV glycoprotein E combined with a liposomal-based adjuvant designed to activate T helper 1 responses.[36] The vaccine has shown a remarkable response in all age groups studied, with a reported reduction of HZ by more than 95%, which is far higher than the Zostavax vaccine. However, these promising results require some caution when considering use in individuals with autoimmune or inflammatory diseases. Although the risks of live-virus administration are not present with the subunit vaccine, there is a potential concern about the use of a strong adjuvant in the autoimmune disease population and the possibility of inducing a flare in underlying disease. Both localized and systemic adverse events were increased in vaccine recipients compared with those receiving placebo in the recently published trial, and it is unknown how this, as-yet unlicensed, adjuvant will behave in people with underlying diseases of the immune system.[36,37] Just as with Zostavax, the subunit vaccine needs to be studied carefully in individuals with autoimmune diseases who may or may not be receiving chronic maintenance immunosuppressive therapy in order to better understand the myriad of potential risks in the context of the magnitude of reduction of HZ.

SUMMARY

It is clear that autoimmune diseases carry with them increased risks of HZ, a painful and often debilitating endogenous reactivation of latent VZV. The magnitude of increased risk may vary by underlying autoimmune disease, which may be related to the specific immune dysregulation characteristic of different diseases. In addition to disease, most medications used to control symptoms and prevent progressive damage are themselves immunosuppressive, and may contribute, to some extent, to the increased rates of HZ seen in these populations. Although studies are varied regarding the increased risks imposed by traditional synthetic immunosuppressant medications, TNFi, and other new biologic and small-molecule therapies, some of the most commonly used medications, glucocorticoids, have been shown unequivocally to affect HZ risk in a dose-dependent manner.

Although it makes the most sense to avoid vaccination during times of highly active disease that requires treatment with induction therapies and high doses of glucocorticoids and combination immunotherapy, there are certain risks involved with delaying initiation of therapy or considering a drug holiday solely for the purpose of vaccination. If it is not safe to delay or stop immunosuppressive therapy, strategies need to be used to protect individuals with reasonably controlled disease on maintenance immunosuppression from developing HZ.

Early evidence, based on retrospective cohort studies or a few very small pilot studies, has suggested that the currently available live-attenuated Zostavax vaccine has a diminished, but still measurable, immune response and reduction of HZ. Furthermore, there have not been significant safety signals that would preclude further carefully controlled studies of vaccination in patients with SLE or RA. Data from larger prospective studies are critical in order to mitigate risk of HZ in these high-risk populations. Furthermore, as alternatives to live-virus vaccination become increasingly available, these vaccines need to be studied head to head with Zostavax to identify the option with the least risk and highest chance of reducing HZ disease burden. In addition, there is good evidence to suggest that young people with autoimmune disease have rates of HZ that equal or exceed the rates in individuals for whom vaccination is recommended (immunocompetent adults $\geq$50 years old), and it is imperative that studies of HZ vaccination include this population of younger adults for whom no vaccine options are currently available.

REFERENCES

1. Centers for Disease Control and Prevention (CDC). Prevention of herpes zoster: recommendations of the Advisory Committee on Immunization Practices (ACIP). MMWR Recomm Rep 2008;57(RR-5):1–30.

2. Galea SA, Sweet A, Beninger P, et al. The safety profile of varicella vaccine: a 10-year review. J Infect Dis 2008;197:S165–9.

3. Levin MJ, Oxman MN, Zhang JH, et al. Varicella-zoster virus-specific immune responses in elderly recipients of a herpes zoster vaccine. J Infect Dis 2008;197: 825–35.

4. Yawn BP, Sakkier P, Wollan PC, et al. A population-based study of the incidence and complication rates of herpes zoster before zoster vaccine introduction. Mayo Clin Proc 2007;82:1341–9.

5. Leung J, Harpaz R, Molinari NA, et al. Herpes zoster incidence among insured persons in the United States, 1993-2006: evaluation of impact of varicella vaccination. Clin Infect Dis 2011;52:332–40.

6. Klein NP, Holmes TH, Sharp MA, et al. Variability and gender differences in memory T cell immunity to varicella-zoster virus in healthy adults. Vaccine 2006;24: 5913–8.

7. Arvin AM. Humor and cellular immunity to varicella-zoster virus: an overview. J Infect Dis 2008;197(Suppl 2):S58–60.

8. Bruer J, Schmid DS, Gershon AA. Use and limitations of varicella-zoster virus-specific serological testing to evaluate breakthrough disease in vaccines and to screen for susceptibility to varicella. J Infect Dis 2008;197(Suppl 2):S147–51.

9. Sadaoka K, Okamoto S, Gomi Y, et al. Measurement of varicella-zoster virus (VZV)-specific cell-mediated immunity: comparison between VZV skin test and

interferon-gamma enzyme-linked immunospot assay. J Infect Dis 2008;198: 1327–33.

10. Chakravarty EF. Viral infection and reactivation in autoimmune diseases. Arthritis Rheum 2008;58:2949–57.

11. Park HB, Kim KC, Park JH, et al. Association of reduced CD4 T cell responses specific to varicella zoster virus with high incidence of herpes zoster in patients with systemic lupus erythematosus. J Rheumatol 2004;31:2151–5.

12. Pope JE, Krizova A, Ouimet JM, et al. Close association of herpes zoster reactivation and systemic lupus erythematosus (SLE) diagnosis: case-control study of patients with SLE or noninflammatory musculoskeletal disorders. J Rheumatol 2004;31:274–9.

13. Wolfe F, Michaud K, Chakravarty EF. Rates and predictors of herpes zoster in patients with rheumatoid arthritis and non-inflammatory musculoskeletal disorders. Rheumatology 2006;45:1370–5.

14. Ishikawa O, Abe M, Miyachi Y. Herpes zoster in Japanese patients with systemic lupus erythematosus. Clin Exp Dermatol 1999;24:327–8.

15. Manzi S, Kuller LH, Kutzer J, et al. Herpes zoster in systemic lupus erythematosus. J Rheumatol 1995;22:1254–8.

16. Kahl LE. Herpes zoster infections in systemic lupus erythematosus: risk factors and outcome. J Rheumatol 1994;21:84–6.

17. Moutsopoulos HM, Gallagher JD, Decker JL, et al. Herpes zoster in patients with systemic lupus erythematosus. Arthritis Rheum 1978;21:789–802.

18. Chakravarty EF, Michaud K, Katz R, et al. Increased incidence of herpes zoster among patients with systemic lupus erythematosus. Lupus 2013;22:238–44.

19. Chen HH, Chen YM, Chen TJ, et al. Risk of herpes zoster in patients with systemic lupus erythematosus: a three-year follow-up study using a nationwide population-based cohort. Clinics (Sao Paulo) 2011;66:1177–82.

20. Hata A, Kuniyoshi M, Ohkusa Y. Risk of herpes zoster inpatients with underlying diseases: a retrospective hospital-based cohort study. Infection 2011;39:537–44.

21. Borba EF, Ribeiro AC, Martin P, et al. Incidence, risk factors, and outcomes of herpes zoster in systemic lupus erythematosus. J Clin Rheumatol 2010;16:119–22.

22. Yun H, Yang S, Chen L, et al. Risk of herpes zoster in auto-immune and inflammatory diseases: implications for vaccination. Arthritis Rheumatol 2016;68(9): 2328–37.

23. Lee PP, Lee TL, Ho MH, et al. Herpes zoster in juvenile-onset lupus erythematosus: incidence, clinical characteristics and risk factors. Pediatr Infect Dis J 2006; 25:728–32.

24. Hu SC, Yen FL, Wang TN, et al. Immunosuppressive medication use and risk of herpes zoster (HZ) in patients with systemic lupus erythematosus (SLE): a nationwide case-control study. J Am Acad Dermatol 2016;75:49–58.

25. Cogman AR, Chakravarty EF. The case for Zostavax vaccination in systemic lupus erythematosus. Vaccine 2013;31:3640–3.

26. Chen SY, Suaya JA, Li Q, et al. Incidence of herpes zoster in patients with altered immune function. Infection 2014;42:325–34.

27. Guthridge JM, Cogman A, Merrill JT, et al. Herpes zoster vaccination in SLE: a pilot study of immunogenicity. J Rheumatol 2013;40:1875–80.

28. Pappas DA, Hooper MM, Kremer JM, et al. Herpes zoster reactivation in patients with rheumatoid arthritis: analysis of disease characteristics and disease-modifying antirheumatic drugs. Arthritis Care Res 2015;67:1671–8.

29. Yun H, Xie F, Delzell E, et al. Risks of herpes zoster in patients with rheumatoid arthritis according to biologic-disease modifying therapy. Arthritis Care Res 2015;67:731–6.

30. Segan J, Staples MP, March L, et al. Risk factors for herpes zoster in rheumatoid arthritis patients: the role of tumor necrosis factor-a inhibitors. Intern Med J 2015; 45:310–8.

31. Ramiro S, Gaujoux-Viala C, Nam JL, et al. Safety of synthetic and biological DMARDs: a systematic literature review informing the 2013 update of the EULAR recommendations for the management of rheumatoid arthritis. Ann Rheum Dis 2014;73:529–35.

32. Che H, Lukas C, Morel J, et al. Risk of herpes/herpes zoster during anti-tumor necrosis factor therapy in patients with rheumatoid arthritis. Systematic review and meta-analysis. Joint Bone Spine 2014;81:215–21.

33. Curtis JR, Xie F, Yun H, et al. Real-world comparative risks of herpes virus infections in tofacitinib and biologic-treated patients with rheumatoid arthritis. Ann Rheum Dis 2016;75(10):1843–7.

34. Winthrop KL, Yamanaka H, Valdez H, et al. Herpes Zoster and tofacitinib therapy in patients with rheumatoid arthritis. Arthritis Rheumatol 2014;66:2675–84.

35. Oxman MN, Levin JM, Johnson GR, et al. A vaccine to prevent herpes zoster and postherpetic neuralgia in older adults. N Engl J Med 2005;352:2271–84.

36. Zhang J, Xie F, Delzell E, et al. Association between vaccination for herpes zoster and risk of herpes zoster infection among older patients with selected immune-mediated diseases. JAMA 2012;308:43–9.

37. Cheetham TC, March SM, Tseng HF, et al. Risk of herpes zoster and disseminated varicella zoster in patients taking immunosuppressant drugs at the time of zoster vaccination. Mayo Clin Proc 2015;90:865–73.

38. Wasan SK, Zullow S, Berg A, et al. Herpes zoster vaccine response in inflammatory bowel disease patients on low-dose immunosuppression. Inflamm Bowel Dis 2016;22:1391–9.

39. Safety and Effectiveness Study of the Live Zoster Vaccine in Anti-TNF Users (VERVE). ClinicalTrials.gov identifier: NCT02538757. Available at: https://clinicaltrials.gov/ct2/show/NCT02538757?term=verve&rank=2. Accessed July 25, 2016.

40. Arnold N, Messaoudi I. Herpes zoster and the search for an effective vaccine. Clin Exp Immunol 2016. http://dx.doi.org/10.1111/cei.12809.

41. Lal H, Cunningham AL, Godeaux O, et al. Efficacy of an adjuvanted herpes zoster subunit vaccine in older adults. N Engl J Med 2015;372:2087–96.

Hepatitis C Virus Infection and Rheumatic Diseases

The Impact of Direct-Acting Antiviral Agents

Patrice Cacoub, MD[a,b,c,d,*], Cloé Commarmond, MD[a,b,c,d],
David Sadoun, MD, PhD[a,b,c,d], Anne Claire Desbois, MD[a,b,c,d]

KEYWORDS

- Hepatitis C (HCV) • Rheumatic disorders • Arthralgia • Arthritis • Vasculitis
- Sicca syndrome • Direct-acting antiviral agents (DAA) • Treatment

KEY POINTS

- Hepatitis C virus infection is associated with many extrahepatic manifestations, including rheumatic disorders such as arthralgia, myalgia, cryoglobulinemia vasculitis, and sicca syndrome.
- The treatment of hepatitis C virus infection has long been based on interferon alfa, which was contraindicated in many autoimmune/inflammatory disorders.
- The emergence of new oral interferon-free combinations now offers an opportunity for patients infected with hepatitis C virus with extrahepatic manifestations, including autoimmune/inflammatory disorders, to be cured with a short treatment duration and a low risk of side effects.

Approximately 130 million to 170 million people are infected with hepatitis C virus (HCV) worldwide. The HCV induces severe morbidity and mortality mainly caused by liver complications (cirrhosis, hepatocellular carcinoma). Shortly after HCV discovery in the early 1990s, this chronic viral infection was recognized to induce many

Conflict of Interest: P. Cacoub has received consultancies, honoraria, advisory board, or speakers' fees from Abbvie, AstraZeneca, Bayer, Boehringer Ingelheim, Gilead, GlaxoSmithKline, Janssen, Merck Sharp and Dohme, Pfizer, Roche, Servier, and Vifor. A.C. Desbois has received speakers' fees from Gilead. C. Commarmond has no conflicts of interest. D. Saadoun has received speakers' fees from Gilead.
Financial support: None.
[a] Inflammation-Immunopathology-Biotherapy Department (DHU i2B), Sorbonne Universités, UPMC Université Paris 06, UMR 7211, Paris F-75005, France; [b] INSERM, UMR_S 959, Paris F-75013, France; [c] CNRS, FRE3632, Paris F-75005, France; [d] Groupe Hospitalier Pitié-Salpêtrière, Department of Internal Medicine and Clinical Immunology, Hôpital Pitié-Salpêtrière, AP-HP, 83 boulevard de l'hôpital, Paris F-75013, France
* Corresponding author. Department of Internal Medicine and Clinical Immunology, Hôpital Pitié-Salpêtrière, AP-HP, 83 boulevard de l'hôpital, Paris F-75013, France.
E-mail address: patrice.cacoub@aphp.fr

extrahepatic manifestations. Large studies have highlighted increased HCV-related morbidity and mortality caused by cryoglobulinemia vasculitis, B-cell non-Hodgkin lymphoma, arthralgia, myalgia, sicca syndrome, as well as cardiovascular diseases, type 2 diabetes and insulin resistance, and neurocognitive dysfunction.[1,2] Interferon alfa (IFN) has long been the cornerstone of antiviral combinations in patients infected with HCV with a low rate of efficacy and a poor tolerance. In addition, use of IFN was associated with high rates of severe adverse events. In patients infected by HCV and with autoimmune/inflammatory rheumatic diseases, IFN was either contraindicated or reported to induce a flare of the disease. Recently, new direct-acting antiviral (DAA) IFN-free treatments led to HCV cure in most (>90%) patients with a good safety profile (severe adverse events <5%) and a short duration (12 weeks). This article focuses on the main rheumatologic diseases associated with chronic HCV infection, and the impact of DAAs on such extrahepatic manifestations.

HEPATITIS C VIRUS AND JOINT MANIFESTATIONS
Arthralgia/Myalgia

Arthralgia is reported in 6% to 20% of patients infected with HCV.[3–5] It usually involves large joints, sometimes with effusion, and is bilateral and symmetric. Arthralgia most frequently involve fingers, knees, and back.[6] Arthralgia is significantly more frequent in patients with cryoglobulinemia vasculitis compared with those without vasculitis (28% vs 23% respectively).[3] The presentation may mimic a rheumatoid arthritis. The frequent positivity of a rheumatoid factor activity in patients infected with HCV also leads to misdiagnosis. Smoking and a previous diagnosis of arthritis are independent risk factors for self-reported joint pain (odds ratio [OR], 5 and 4.25, respectively). Myalgia is less common, affecting about 2% to 5% of patients with HCV.[3,5] Arthritis, unrelated to mixed cryoglobulinemia, is less common (<5% of patient), involving small joints associated with carpal tunnel syndrome and palmar tenosynovitis.

Hepatitis C Virus Mixed Cryoglobulinemia Vasculitis

Mixed cryoglobulinemia vasculitis (CryoVas) is an immune complex small vessel vasculitis involving mainly the skin, the joints, the peripheral nerve system, and the kidneys.[1,2] Cryoglobulinemia is defined by the presence of circulating immunoglobulins that precipitate at cold temperatures and dissolve with rewarming. CryoVas is related to HCV infection in 70% to 80% of cases, mostly associated with a type II immunoglobulin (Ig) M kappa mixed cryoglobulin. In contrast, 50% to 60% of patients infected with HCV produce a mixed cryoglobulin that leads to CryoVas in 15% of cases. Main symptoms include asthenia, purpura, arthralgia, myalgia, peripheral neuropathy, and glomerulonephritis.[7,8] In a large cohort of patients with HCV-CryoVas, baseline factors associated with a poor prognosis were the presence of severe liver fibrosis (hazard ratio [HR], 5.31), central nervous system involvement (HR, 2.74), kidney involvement (HR, 1.91), and heart involvement (HR, 4.2).[9] Arthralgia is reported in 40% to 80% of patients infected with HCV and positive for a mixed cryoglobulin.[10–12] Joint pains are bilateral, symmetric, nondeforming, and involve mainly knees and hands, less commonly elbows and ankles. Rheumatoid factor (RF) activity is found in 70% to 80% of patients with CryoVas, not correlated with the occurrence of joint disease. Anti–cyclic citrullinated peptide (anti-CCP) antibodies are usually absent in patients with HCV. Clinically or on imaging, there is no evidence of joint destruction. Of note, some clinical features might be confusing for clinicians, because IFN treatment used for HCV may lead to exacerbation of arthralgia and myalgia. Sometimes it used to be difficult to distinguish vasculitis flares and side effects of IFN-based treatments.

Sicca Syndrome

Sicca symptoms of either the mouth or eyes have been reported in 10% to 30% of patients infected with HCV. Less than 5% of patients with a defined Sjögren syndrome are HCV positive.[10] In a recent literature review, Younossi and colleagues[13] reported a sicca syndrome prevalence of 11.9% in patients with HCV, with a risk ratio for sicca syndrome of 2.29 in patients infected with HCV compared with uninfected patients. However, the criteria for Sjögren syndrome diagnosis were based on clinical questionnaire in some studies and were not well detailed. Although sicca symptoms are very common in patients infected with HCV, a characterized Sjögren syndrome defined by the presence of anti-SSA or anti-SSB antibodies and a typical salivary gland histology is uncommon. A large cohort study of 137 patients with a definite Sjögren syndrome (1993 international criteria) compared patients with HCV infection with those with a primary form. Patients with HCV-associated Sjögren syndrome were older; more frequently male; and more frequently presented a vasculitis, a peripheral neuropathy, and a neoplasia. They also had a different biological pattern; that is, they more frequently had a positive RF test, a cryoglobulinemia, and less frequently anti-SSA or SSB antibodies.[14,15] Only 23% of patients with HCV-associated Sjögren syndrome had positive anti-extractable nuclear antigen. The detection of HCV RNA and HCV core antigen in epithelial cells of patients with HCV-associated Sjögren syndrome and the development of Sjögren syndrome–like exocrinopathy in transgenic mice carrying the HCV envelope genes support the possibility of a direct impact of HCV on the development of sialadenitis.[16,17]

Fibromyalgia and Fatigue

In a large prospective study, 19% of 1614 patients infected with HCV fulfilled the main diagnostic criteria of fibromyalgia (fatigue, arthralgia, and myalgia).[3] Fatigue, with or without a fibromyalgia, was the most frequent extrahepatic manifestation (35%–67%). Many underlying factors were independently associated with fatigue, such as older age, female gender, the presence of arthralgia/myalgia, as well as neuropsychological factors. In contrast, there was no link with alcohol consumption, HCV genotype or viral load, the presence of a cryoglobulin, and thyroid dysfunction. Of note, after IFN-based treatment, only the group of patients with a sustained virologic response showed a beneficial impact on fatigue. A benefit of treatment on arthralgia/myalgia was found in about 50% of patients, independently of the virologic response.

Production of Autoantibodies

The prevalence of circulating autoantibodies is high in patients with chronic HCV infection, which may cause diagnostic difficulties in patients with rheumatic manifestations.[3,10] The most frequent immunologic abnormalities include mixed cryoglobulins (50%–60%); RF activity (40%); and antinuclear (20%–35%), anticardiolipin (10%–15%), antithyroid (10%), and anti–smooth muscle antibodies (7%).[3,18,19] At least 1 immunologic abnormality is present in up to 53% of patients infected with HCV. The presence of such antibodies (ie, RF, antinuclear, or anticardiolipin) is usually not associated with specific clinical symptoms related to autoimmune disease.[3,20] The most frequent risk factors for the presence of such biological extrahepatic manifestations are the presence of extensive liver fibrosis and older age.[3,19]

Underlying Mechanisms

There are multiple immunologic factors predisposing patients infected with HCV to develop a CryoVas or other systemic rheumatologic manifestations. Chronic stimulation of B cells by HCV directly modulates B-cell and T-cell function and results in polyclonal activation and expansion of B cell–producing IgM with RF activity. There is an expansion of clonal $CD21^{-/low}IgM^+CD27^+$ marginal zone–like B cells,[21] and a decrease of regulatory T cells.[22] In a genome-wide association study, significant associations were identified on chromosome 6.[23] A higher percentage of a particular allele of the promoter of the B cell–activating factor has been shown.[24] In contrast, specific virologic factors (viral load, genotype) have not been identified. Other factors are related to the infection by HCV of peripheral blood mononuclear cells, including peripheral dendritic cells, monocytes, and macrophages.[25] A persistent viral stimulation enhances expression of lymphomagenesis-related genes, particularly the activation-induced cytidine deaminase, which is critical for somatic hypermutation and could lead to polyclonal and, later, monoclonal expansion of B cells.[26] Under this trigger effect, oligoclonal or monoclonal IgM, which share rheumatoid activity, are produced by a permanent clone of B cells that favors the appearance of immune complexes, formed by circulating HCV, anti-HCV polyclonal IgG, and the monoclonal IgM.

IMPACT OF HEPATITIS C VIRUS CHRONIC INFECTION IN PATIENTS WITH RHEUMATOLOGIC DISORDERS
Increased Cardiometabolic-related Morbidity and Mortality

Many chronic autoimmune rheumatic diseases are now well recognized as independent risk factors for major cardiovascular events. Recent data also provide evidence of a strong relationship between HCV infection and major adverse cardiovascular events. Such risk has been shown to be higher in patients infected with HCV compared with controls without HCV, independently of the severity of the liver disease or the common cardiovascular risk factors. Patients with HCV chronic infection have an increased prevalence of carotid atherosclerosis and increased intima-media thickness compared with healthy controls or patients with hepatitis B or nonalcoholic steatohepatitis. Active chronic HCV infection seems to be an independent risk factor for ischemic cerebrovascular accidents and ischemic heart disease.[27] For example, Maruyama and colleagues[28] reported an improvement in the myocardial perfusion defect in patients who were cured from HCV infection after IFN-based treatment, whereas relapsers showed worsening. Successful IFN-based therapy showed a beneficial impact on the cardiovascular risk, underlining the tight link between HCV and the occurrence of cardiovascular events.[29–31] Consistently, HCV infection has been associated with higher rates of diabetes mellitus and insulin resistance compared with healthy volunteers and patients with hepatitis B. In addition, glucose abnormalities in patients with HCV are associated with poor liver outcomes, defined by advanced liver fibrosis, lack of sustained virologic response to IFN-based treatment, and a higher risk of hepatocellular carcinoma development.[32–35] In the context of chronic inflammatory rheumatologic disorders, which already lead to an increased cardiovascular risk (related to chronic inflammation), the presence of HCV infection should be taken into account to assess the global cardiovascular risk.

Rheumatologic Impact

Studies analyzing the impact of HCV infection on the prognosis of patients with chronic inflammatory rheumatologic disorders are scarce. In a recent prospective cohort of US veterans, HCV-positive patients reported higher pain scores, had higher tender joint counts, and higher patient global scores contributing to higher disease activity score (DAS)28 scores, after adjustment for age, gender, race, smoking status, and days from enrollment.[36] After further adjustments for differences in the use of methotrexate, prednisone, and anti-TNF therapies, DAS28 scores remained significantly higher in HCV-positive patients over all study visits. There was no difference in physician-reported outcomes (swollen joints or physician global scores). After adjusting for age, gender, and race, HCV-positive patients were more likely to use prednisone (OR, 1.41) and anti-TNF therapies (OR, 1.51), and far less likely to use methotrexate (OR, 0.27).[36]

TREATMENT OF HEPATITIS C VIRUS INFECTION
Before the Era of Direct-acting Antiviral Combinations

The cornerstone of HCV-CryoVas therapy is the capacity of treatments to achieve a sustained virologic response. Introduced in the early 1980s as a monotherapy, IFN was found to be both poorly tolerated and poorly effective with virologic cure (sustained virologic response [SVR]) in less than 10%. With pegylated formulations of IFN (Peg-IFN) optimizing its pharmacokinetics and combination with ribavirin for 48 weeks or longer, SVR rates increased to about 50%. During the decade 2000 to 2010, Mazzaro and colleagues[37] first reported sustained clinical and virologic response in 44% of patients with HCV-CryoVas treated with Peg-IFN plus ribavirin for 12 months. Saadoun and colleagues[38] reported that the combination of Peg-IFN plus ribavirin compared with IFN plus ribavirin showed higher rates of complete clinical (67.5% vs 56.2%) and virologic (62.5% vs 53.1%) responses, regardless of HCV genotype and viral load. An early virologic response was associated with a complete clinical response (OR, 3.53; 95% confidence interval [CI], 1.18, 10.59), whereas a glomerular filtration rate less than 70 mL/min was a negative predictor (OR, 0.18; 95% CI, 0.05, 0.67). However, the safety profile was not satisfactory and such therapies often led to many severe adverse events, such as severe cytopenia, disabling fatigue, fever, and depression. In addition, fatigue, arthralgia, and myalgia were frequently reported, which is a particular concern in rheumatology patients in whom distinguishing drug side effect from underlying disease was often difficult.[39] Although nonspecific arthralgia has been reported, some investigators have published rare cases of rheumatoid arthritis occurrence with anti-CCP antibodies after IFN-based treatment despite HCV cure.[40,41] Consistently, other autoimmune exacerbations, such as Sjögren syndrome and systemic lupus erythematosus, have been reported after IFN treatments.[42] In the context of CryoVas, it has been reported cases of peripheral neuropathy induced or flared by IFN-based treatment.[43]

THE ERA OF DIRECT-ACTING ANTIVIRAL COMBINATIONS

The beginning of the new era was characterized by the development of the first 2 DAA agents: boceprevir and telaprevir. In combination with Peg-IFN and ribavirin, these first-generation HCV protease inhibitors significantly improved the efficacy of antiviral combination, leading to approximately 70% SVR rate in genotype 1 HCV infection. However, these agents worsened the toxicity of IFN-based treatments, which limited their use in all patients with HCV as well as in patients with rheumatic diseases.[15] In a prospective cohort of patients with HCV treated with boceprevir, the SVR rate was lower in cryoglobulinemic patients than in those without mixed cryoglobulinemia (23.8% vs 70% respectively; $P = .01$),[44] although the latter had more risk factors of treatment failure (severe liver fibrosis). The boceprevir-based treatment allowed improvement of symptoms on undetectable viremia and resulted in cryocrit disappearance in 86% of patients. However, symptoms reappeared after virologic breakthrough.[44] In another prospective study, telaprevir or boceprevir showed complete clinical response and SVR at week 24 in 67% of patients. However, serious adverse events occurred in 46.6% of patients, mostly in patients with baseline severe liver fibrosis and a low platelet count.[44,45]

More recently, new all-oral, IFN-free, as well as ribavirin-free regimens have been approved. They are characterized by a dramatic efficacy leading to cure rates of 90% to 100% in all HCV genotypes, with minimal side effects and short duration (12–24 weeks).[46,47] Even in difficult-to-treat populations, including cirrhotic and previously treated patients, IFN-free DAA regimens have been reported to be very efficient. Numerous large prospective studies have been published with different DAA combinations, such as simeprevir plus sofosbuvir,[48] sofosbuvir plus daclatasvir with/without ribavirin, or sofosbuvir plus ledipasvir, showing high antiviral potency (>90% SVR rates in both cirrhotic and treatment-experienced patients whatever the stage of fibrosis).[49] Although such treatments remain expensive, they now offer a therapeutic revolution for patients infected with HCV, particularly those with rheumatic diseases in whom IFN-based treatment has failed or was not well tolerated.

For the treatment of HCV-CryoVas, the VASCUVALDIC study enrolled 24 patients (median age, 56.5 years; 54% male; 50% cirrhotic) who received sofosbuvir plus ribavirin for 24 weeks.[12] Seven patients also received immunosuppressive therapy; that is, rituximab, corticosteroids, and plasmapheresis. Eighty-seven percent of patients were complete clinical responders and SVR was obtained in 74% of patients at week12 posttreatment. Of note, the complete clinical response was very rapid because it was noted at on-treatment week 12 in two-thirds of patients. Kidney involvement with membranoproliferative glomerulonephritis improved in 4 out of 5 patients. Only 2 (8%) serious adverse events were observed. Sise and colleagues[50] reported a retrospective case series of 12 patients with HCV-CryoVas (median age, 61 years; 58% male; 50% cirrhotic) treated with sofosbuvir plus simeprevir (n = 8) or sofosbuvir plus ribavirin (n = 4). Seven patients had evidence of renal involvement, including 5 patients with membranoproliferative glomerulonephritis. Four patients received rituximab concurrent with DAA therapy. An SVR at posttreatment week 12 was achieved in 83% of patients. Cryoglobulin levels decreased in most patients, with a median decrease from 1.5% to 0.5%, and disappeared in 4 out of 9 cases. Only 2 (17%) patients experienced serious adverse events. The Italian experience was recently reported in 37 patients with HCV-CryoVas who received DAAs.[51] Ten percent of patients also received immunosuppressants. A response on CryoVas symptoms was defined as complete in 18 (49%) and partial in 13 (35%), whereas no response was noted in 6 (16%) patients.

Despite the unquestionable evidence of a viral cause and the obvious efficacy of antiviral treatments, immunosuppression remains a major treatment in patients with HCV-CryoVas in cases of severe presentation (renal, digestive, or cardiac involvements) or in patients with failure or contraindication to antiviral treatment. Rituximab (a monoclonal anti–CD20 antibody) targets activated B cells, which are responsible for cryoglobulin production and eventually CryoVas lesions. Randomized controlled trials showed that rituximab has a better efficacy than conventional immunosuppressive treatments (ie, glucocorticoids, azathioprine, cyclophosphamide, or plasmapheresis) or placebo.[52,53] Two other controlled trials showed that addition of rituximab to Peg-IFN/ribavirin led to a shorter time to clinical remission, better renal response rate, and higher rates of cryoglobulin clearance.[54,55] Of note, paradoxic worsening of vasculitis has also been described after rituximab in such patients. Rituximab may form a complex with IgMk mixed cryoglobulin and lead to severe exacerbation of vasculitis involvements.[56] Considering the very rapid and potent virologic efficacy of new DAA combination and the proven correlation between SVR and clinical response, the exact place of rituximab, plasmapheresis, or other immunosuppressive drugs remains to be defined.[56] Other treatments for CryoVas have a limited place. Corticosteroids, used alone or in addition to IFN, did not favorably affect the response of HCV-CryoVas manifestations in controlled studies.[57] Plasmapheresis, which offers the advantage of removing the pathogenic cryoglobulins from the circulation, should be considered for rapidly progressive glomerulonephritis or life-threatening involvements. Immunosuppressive therapy is usually needed in association with plasma exchange in order to avoid the rebound increase in cryoglobulin serum level seen after discontinuation of apheresis. When used in combination with HCV treatment, plasmapheresis did not modify the virologic response if IFN was given after each plasma exchange session.[58] There are no available data to date with DAA.

The impact of new DAAs on other rheumatologic manifestations (ie, arthralgia, myalgia, and sicca syndrome) is unknown. For fibromyalgia, Younossi and colleagues[59] recently reported major benefits of sofosbuvir-based DAAs on most patient-reported outcomes, including mental and physical fatigue, at week 12 and week 24 posttreatment. A benefit of DAAs was also suggested on cerebral magnetic resonance signal in basal ganglia correlated with the virologic response.[60]

In conclusion, HCV chronic infection, apart from its liver-related complications, is frequently associated with clinical and biological rheumatologic manifestations, such as arthralgia, myalgia, cryoglobulinemia vasculitis, sicca syndrome, and the production of autoantibodies. Treatment of HCV has long been based on IFN, excluding most patients with rheumatisms because of the poor efficacy, high rates of side effects, and the risk of exacerbation of autoimmune and rheumatic disorders. The emergence of new oral IFN-free combinations now offers the opportunity for patients infected with HCV with extrahepatic manifestations such as rheumatic disorders to be cured with a low risk of side effects and a short treatment duration.

REFERENCES

1. Cacoub P, Gragnani L, Comarmond C, et al. Extrahepatic manifestations of chronic hepatitis C virus infection. Dig Liver Dis 2014;46(Suppl 5):S165–73.

2. Ferri C, Sebastiani M, Giuggioli D, et al. Hepatitis C virus syndrome: a constellation of organ- and non-organ specific autoimmune disorders, B-cell non-Hodgkin's lymphoma, and cancer. World J Hepatol 2015;7:327–43.

3. Cacoub P, Poynard T, Ghillani P, et al. Extrahepatic manifestations of chronic hepatitis C. MULTIVIRC Group. Multidepartment Virus C. Arthritis Rheum 1999;42: 2204–12.

4. Cheng Z, Zhou B, Shi X, et al. Extrahepatic manifestations of chronic hepatitis C virus infection: 297 cases from a tertiary medical center in Beijing, China. Chin Med J (Engl) 2014;127:1206–10.

5. Mohammed RHA, ElMakhzangy HI, Gamal A, et al. Prevalence of rheumatologic manifestations of chronic hepatitis C virus infection among Egyptians. Clin Rheumatol 2010;29:1373–80.

6. Ogdie A, Pang WG, Forde KA, et al. Prevalence and risk factors for patient-reported joint pain among patients with HIV/hepatitis C coinfection, hepatitis C monoinfection, and HIV monoinfection. BMC Musculoskelet Disord 2015;16:93.

7. Landau D-A, Scerra S, Sene D, et al. Causes and predictive factors of mortality in a cohort of patients with hepatitis C virus-related cryoglobulinemic vasculitis treated with antiviral therapy. J Rheumatol 2010;37:615–21.

8. Ferri C, Sebastiani M, Giuggioli D, et al. Mixed cryoglobulinemia: demographic, clinical, and serologic features and survival in 231 patients. Semin Arthritis Rheum 2004;33:355–74.

9. Terrier B, Semoun O, Saadoun D, et al. Prognostic factors in patients with hepatitis C virus infection and systemic vasculitis. Arthritis Rheum 2011;63:1748–57.

10. Cacoub P, Renou C, Rosenthal E, et al. Extrahepatic manifestations associated with hepatitis C virus infection. A prospective multicenter study of 321 patients. The GERMIVIC. Groupe d'Etude et de Recherche en Medecine Interne et Maladies Infectieuses sur le Virus de l'Hepatite C. Medicine (Baltimore) 2000;79: 47–56.

11. Lee YH, Ji JD, Yeon JE, et al. Cryoglobulinaemia and rheumatic manifestations in patients with hepatitis C virus infection. Ann Rheum Dis 1998;57:728–31.

12. Saadoun D, Thibault V, Si Ahmed SN, et al. Sofosbuvir plus ribavirin for hepatitis C virus-associated cryoglobulinaemia vasculitis: VASCUVALDIC study. Ann Rheum Dis 2016;75(10):1777–82.

13. Younossi Z, Park H, Henry L, et al. Extra-hepatic manifestations of hepatitis C—a meta-analysis of prevalence, quality of life, and economic burden. Gastroenterology 2016;150(7):1599–608.

14. Brito-Zerón P, Gheitasi H, Retamozo S, et al. How hepatitis C virus modifies the immunological profile of Sjögren syndrome: analysis of 783 patients. Arthritis Res Ther 2015;17:250.

15. Ramos-Casals M, Loustaud-Ratti V, De Vita S, et al. Sjögren syndrome associated with hepatitis C virus: a multicenter analysis of 137 cases. Medicine (Baltimore) 2005;84:81–9.

16. Arrieta JJ, Rodríguez-Iñigo E, Ortiz-Movilla N, et al. In situ detection of hepatitis C virus RNA in salivary glands. Am J Pathol 2001;158:259–64.

17. Koike K, Moriya K, Ishibashi K, et al. Sialadenitis histologically resembling Sjogren syndrome in mice transgenic for hepatitis C virus envelope genes. Proc Natl Acad Sci U S A 1997;94:233–6.

18. Khairy M, El-Raziky M, El-Akel W, et al. Serum autoantibodies positivity prevalence in patients with chronic HCV and impact on pegylated interferon and ribavirin treatment response. Liver Int 2013;33:1504–9.

19. Hsieh M-Y, Dai C-Y, Lee L-P, et al. Antinuclear antibody is associated with a more advanced fibrosis and lower RNA levels of hepatitis C virus in patients with chronic hepatitis C. J Clin Pathol 2008;61:333–7.

20. Himoto T, Masaki T. Extrahepatic manifestations and autoantibodies in patients with hepatitis C virus infection. Clin Dev Immunol 2012;2012:871401.

21. Terrier B, Joly F, Vazquez T, et al. Expansion of functionally anergic CD21-/low marginal zone-like B cell clones in hepatitis C virus infection-related autoimmunity. J Immunol 2011;187:6550–63.

22. Saadoun D, Rosenzwajg M, Joly F, et al. Regulatory T-cell responses to low-dose interleukin-2 in HCV-induced vasculitis. N Engl J Med 2011;365:2067–77.

23. Zignego AL, Wojcik GL, Cacoub P, et al. Genome-wide association study of hepatitis C virus- and cryoglobulin-related vasculitis. Genes Immun 2014;15:500–5.

24. Gragnani L, Piluso A, Giannini C, et al. Genetic determinants in hepatitis C virus-associated mixed cryoglobulinemia: role of polymorphic variants of BAFF promoter and Fcγ receptors. Arthritis Rheum 2011;63:1446–51.

25. Caussin-Schwemling C, Schmitt C, Stoll-Keller F. Study of the infection of human blood derived monocyte/macrophages with hepatitis C virus in vitro. J Med Virol 2001;65:14–22.

26. Muramatsu M, Kinoshita K, Fagarasan S, et al. Class switch recombination and hypermutation require activation-induced cytidine deaminase (AID), a potential RNA editing enzyme. Cell 2000;102:553–63.

27. Domont F, Cacoub P. Chronic hepatitis C virus infection, a new cardiovascular risk factor? Liver Int 2016;36:621–7.

28. Maruyama S, Koda M, Oyake N, et al. Myocardial injury in patients with chronic hepatitis C infection. J Hepatol 2013;58:11–5.

29. Hsu Y-H, Hung P-H, Muo C-H, et al. Interferon-based treatment of hepatitis C virus infection reduces all-cause mortality in patients with end-stage renal disease: an 8-year nationwide cohort study in Taiwan. Medicine (Baltimore) 2015;94: e2113.

30. Hsu Y-C, Lin J-T, Ho HJ, et al. Antiviral treatment for hepatitis C virus infection is associated with improved renal and cardiovascular outcomes in diabetic patients. Hepatology 2014;59:1293–302.

31. Hsu C-S, Kao J-H, Chao Y-C, et al. Interferon-based therapy reduces risk of stroke in chronic hepatitis C patients: a population-based cohort study in Taiwan. Aliment Pharmacol Ther 2013;38:415–23.

32. Elkrief L, Chouinard P, Bendersky N, et al. Diabetes mellitus is an independent prognostic factor for major liver-related outcomes in patients with cirrhosis and chronic hepatitis C. Hepatology 2014;60:823–31.

33. Huang Y-W, Yang S-S, Fu S-C, et al. Increased risk of cirrhosis and its decompensation in chronic hepatitis C patients with new-onset diabetes: A nationwide cohort study. Hepatology 2014;60:807–14.

34. Hung C-H, Lee C-M, Wang J-H, et al. Impact of diabetes mellitus on incidence of hepatocellular carcinoma in chronic hepatitis C patients treated with interferon-based antiviral therapy. Int J Cancer 2011;128:2344–52.

35. Eslam M, Aparcero R, Kawaguchi T, et al. Meta-analysis: insulin resistance and sustained virological response in hepatitis C. Aliment Pharmacol Ther 2011;34: 297–305.

36. Patel R, Mikuls TR, Richards JS, et al. Disease characteristics and treatment patterns in veterans with rheumatoid arthritis and concomitant hepatitis C infection. Arthritis Care Res 2015;67:467–74.

37. Mazzaro C, Zorat F, Caizzi M, et al. Treatment with peg-interferon alfa-2b and ribavirin of hepatitis C virus-associated mixed cryoglobulinemia: a pilot study. J Hepatol 2005;42:632–8.

38. Saadoun D, Resche-Rigon M, Thibault V, et al. Antiviral therapy for hepatitis C virus–associated mixed cryoglobulinemia vasculitis: a long-term followup study. Arthritis Rheum 2006;54:3696–706.

39. Cacoub P, Comarmond C, Domont F, et al. Cryoglobulinemia vasculitis. Am J Med 2015;128:950–5.

40. Yang D, Arkfeld D, Fong T-L. Development of anti-CCP-positive rheumatoid arthritis following pegylated interferon-α2a treatment for chronic hepatitis C infection. J Rheumatol 2010;37:1777.

41. Cacopardo B, Benanti F, Pinzone MR, et al. Rheumatoid arthritis following PEG-interferon-alfa-2a plus ribavirin treatment for chronic hepatitis C: a case report and review of the literature. BMC Res Notes 2013;6:437.

42. Onishi S, Nagashima T, Kimura H, et al. Systemic lupus erythematosus and Sjögren's syndrome induced in a case by interferon-alpha used for the treatment of hepatitis C. Lupus 2010;19:753–5.

43. Stübgen J-P. Interferon alpha and neuromuscular disorders. J Neuroimmunol 2009;207:3–17.

44. Gragnani L, Fabbrizzi A, Triboli E, et al. Triple antiviral therapy in hepatitis C virus infection with or without mixed cryoglobulinaemia: A prospective, controlled pilot study. Dig Liver Dis 2014;46:833–7.

45. Saadoun D, Resche Rigon M, Pol S, et al. PegIFNα/ribavirin/protease inhibitor combination in severe hepatitis C virus-associated mixed cryoglobulinemia vasculitis. J Hepatol 2015;62:24–30.

46. Afdhal N, Zeuzem S, Kwo P, et al. Ledipasvir and sofosbuvir for untreated HCV genotype 1 infection. N Engl J Med 2014;370:1889–98.

47. Sulkowski MS, Gardiner DF, Rodriguez-Torres M, et al. Daclatasvir plus sofosbuvir for previously treated or untreated chronic HCV infection. N Engl J Med 2014; 370:211–21.

48. Sulkowski MS, Vargas HE, Di Bisceglie AM, et al. Effectiveness of simeprevir plus sofosbuvir, with or without ribavirin, in real-world patients with HCV genotype 1 infection. Gastroenterology 2016;150:419–29.

49. Pol S, Corouge M, Vallet-Pichard A. Daclatasvir-sofosbuvir combination therapy with or without ribavirin for hepatitis C virus infection: from the clinical trials to real life. Hepat Med 2016;8:21–6.

50. Sise ME, Bloom AK, Wisocky J, et al. Treatment of hepatitis C virus associated mixed cryoglobulinemia with direct-acting antiviral agents. Hepatology 2016; 63:408–17.

51. Kondili LA, Weimer LE, Mallano A, et al. HCV-related mixed cryoglobulinemia: data from PITER, a nationwide Italian HCV cohort study. J Hepatol 2016;64:S618.

52. De Vita S, Quartuccio L, Isola M, et al. A randomized controlled trial of rituximab for the treatment of severe cryoglobulinemic vasculitis. Arthritis Rheum 2012;64: 843–53.

53. Sneller MC, Hu Z, Langford CA. A randomized controlled trial of rituximab following failure of antiviral therapy for hepatitis C virus-associated cryoglobulinemic vasculitis. Arthritis Rheum 2012;64:835–42.

54. Saadoun D, Resche Rigon M, Sene D, et al. Rituximab plus Peg-interferon-alpha/ ribavirin compared with Peg-interferon-alpha/ribavirin in hepatitis C-related mixed cryoglobulinemia. Blood 2010;116:326–34 [quiz: 504–5].

55. Dammacco F, Tucci FA, Lauletta G, et al. Pegylated interferon-alpha, ribavirin, and rituximab combined therapy of hepatitis C virus-related mixed cryoglobulinemia: a long-term study. Blood 2010;116:343–53.

56. Sène D, Ghillani-Dalbin P, Amoura Z, et al. Rituximab may form a complex with IgMkappa mixed cryoglobulin and induce severe systemic reactions in patients with hepatitis C virus-induced vasculitis. Arthritis Rheum 2009;60:3848–55.

57. Dammacco F, Sansonno D, Han JH, et al. Natural interferon-alpha versus its combination with 6-methyl-prednisolone in the therapy of type II mixed cryoglobulinemia: a long-term, randomized, controlled study. Blood 1994;84:3336–43.

58. Hausfater P, Cacoub P, Assogba U, et al. Plasma exchange and interferon-alpha pharmacokinetics in patients with hepatitis C virus-associated systemic vasculitis. Nephron 2002;91:627–30.

59. Younossi ZM, Stepanova M, Marcellin P, et al. Treatment with ledipasvir and sofosbuvir improves patient-reported outcomes: results from the ION-1, -2, and -3 clinical trials. Hepatology 2015;61:1798–808.

60. Byrnes V, Miller A, Lowry D, et al. Effects of anti-viral therapy and HCV clearance on cerebral metabolism and cognition. J Hepatol 2012;56:549–56.

Hepatitis B Reactivation in Rheumatic Diseases

Screening and Prevention

Christos Koutsianas, MD[a,b], Konstantinos Thomas, MD[a],
Dimitrios Vassilopoulos, MD[a],*

KEYWORDS

- Hepatitis B • Reactivation • Rheumatic diseases
- Disease-modifying antirheumatic drugs • Biologics • TNF inhibitors • Rituximab
- Tocilizumab • Abatacept

KEY POINTS

- The risk for hepatitis B virus (HBV) reactivation (HBVr) is high for rheumatic patients with chronic infection treated with high-dose corticosteroids (CS), tumor necrosis factor inhibitors, and rituximab (RTX) without antiviral prophylaxis, whereas it seems to be minimal for patients with past HBV infection.
- HBV serologic screening is required for almost all rheumatic patients before immunosuppressive therapies.
- Prophylactic antiviral therapy with the new-generation antivirals, such as entecavir and tenofovir, is required for all patients starting long-term CS and biologics.
- Patients with past HBV infection receiving high-risk therapy, such as RTX, should be screened and monitored by HBV DNA measurements and treated when HBVr is documented.

INTRODUCTION

The risk for hepatitis B virus (HBV) reactivation (HBVr) during immunosuppressive therapy in patients with chronic or less frequently past HBV infection is increasingly recognized today in different disciplines of medicine, including rheumatology.[1,2] HBVr

---

Disclosure Statement: The authors have nothing to disclose.
[a] Joint Rheumatology Program, Clinical Immunology-Rheumatology Unit, 2nd Department of Medicine and Laboratory, National and Kapodistrian University of Athens School of Medicine, Hippokration General Hospital, 114 Vass, Sophias Avenue, Athens 115 27, Greece; [b] Department of Rheumatology, The Dudley Group NHS Foundation Trust, Russells Hall Hospital, Pennsett Road, Dudley DY1 2HQ, West Midlands, UK
* Corresponding author. Joint Rheumatology Program, Clinical Immunology-Rheumatology Unit, 2nd Department of Medicine and Laboratory, Hippokration General Hospital, National and Kapodistrian University of Athens School of Medicine, 114 Vass. Sophias Avenue, Athens 115 27, Greece.
E-mail address: dvassilop@med.uoa.gr

Rheum Dis Clin N Am 43 (2017) 133–149
http://dx.doi.org/10.1016/j.rdc.2016.09.012
0889-857X/17/© 2016 Elsevier Inc. All rights reserved.

during immunosuppressive therapy can range from an asymptomatic increase in HBV DNA levels to fatal hepatic failure. Better screening and monitoring of HBV-infected patients, as well as early management of HBV infection with the last-generation oral antivirals, has greatly improved the outcome of HBVr in this setting. Here the authors review the existing literature on HBVr in rheumatic patients and propose a screening and management algorithm for patients at risk.

EPIDEMIOLOGY OF CHRONIC AND PAST HEPATITIS B VIRUS INFECTION

HBV is a partially double-stranded DNA virus primarily infecting humans through the parenteral route.[3,4] Most chronically infected patients have acquired the virus either perinatally (in areas of high endemicity: >7%) or through horizontal transmission during childhood (in areas of intermediate endemicity: 2%–7%). Exposure during adulthood (through unprotected sexual intercourse, intravenous drug use, or occupational exposure) rarely leads to chronic infection (<5%).[4,5] With the introduction of efficient preventive measures, such as universal vaccination of infants, prevention of perinatal transmission, and vaccination of high-risk adults, several studies have shown a decrease in the incidence of acute HBV infection that is not yet followed by a similar reduction in the sequelae of chronic disease.[6,7]

The prevalence of chronic HBV infection varies worldwide and is highest in sub-Saharan Africa and East Asia (5%–10%) and lowest in Western Europe and North America (<1%).[5] It has to be noted that even in low endemic areas, such as the United States, the prevalence of chronic HBV infection may be significantly higher in specific groups, such as immigrants and institutionalized and incarcerated individuals. A similar geographic variation has been found in the prevalence of resolved HBV infection, with less than 5% of the population in North America having past exposure to the virus,[8] whereas the respective rate exceeds 50% in areas of high endemicity.

Most studies indicate that the rates of chronic and resolved HBV infection in rheumatic patients follow the patterns of the general population. In 2 recent, large, multiethnic, cross-sectional studies in rheumatoid arthritis (RA) and spondyloarthritis,[9,10] the prevalence of chronic HBV infection was estimated at 3.0% and 3.5%, respectively, although percentages up to 12% in some participating countries were recorded.[9,10] Similarly, the prevalence of resolved HBV infection ranged between 13% and 15% in European,[11,12] 25% to 30% in Japanese,[13,14] and 50% in Chinese[15] cohorts of patients with RA.[16]

DIAGNOSIS AND CLASSIFICATION OF HEPATITIS B VIRUS INFECTION

The diagnosis of HBV infection relies mainly on serology (hepatitis B surface antigen [HBsAg], hepatitis B envelope antigen [HBeAg], anti-HBs, anti-HBc [hepatitis B core antibody] and anti-HBe antibodies) and serum HBV DNA levels.[4,5] Serologic tests are used for the differentiation between acute, chronic, or past (resolved) infection, whereas HBV DNA levels are required for distinguishing active chronic hepatitis from the inactive carrier state in chronically infected patients as well as for the detection of occult infection in resolved HBV infection (**Table 1**).

More specifically:

1. *Acute hepatitis B* is characterized by high aminotransferases (alanine aminotransferase [ALT] >10× the upper limit of normal [ULN]) and positive HBsAg and IgM anti-HBc antibodies. These patients are rarely encountered in rheumatology practice.
2. The *chronic HBV infection* definition requires the presence of HBsAg in the serum for greater than 6 months. Most of these patients (70%–80%) are *inactive HBV carriers*

Table 1
Laboratory diagnosis of hepatitis B virus infection

| | | Chronic Infection | | | |
| | | Chronic Hepatitis | | | |
	Acute Hepatitis	HBeAg Positive	HBeAg Negative	Inactive Carrier State	Past (Resolved) Infection
HBsAg	+	+	+	+	−
Anti-HBc (total)	+	+	+	+	+
Anti-HBs	−	−	−	−	±
Anti-HBc IgM	+	−	−	−	−
HBeAg	+	+	−	−	−
Anti-HBe	−	−	+	±	+
ALT	↑↑↑ (usually >10× ULN)	↑	↑	Normal	Normal
HBV DNA	>20,000 IU/mL[a]	>20,000 IU/mL	>2,000 IU/mL	Undetectable or <2,000 IU/mL	Undetectable[b]

Abbreviation: ALT, alanine aminotransferase.
[a] Usually greater than 10^6 IU/mL.
[b] In patients with occult infection, HBV DNA can be detected in the liver or in the serum (<200 IU/mL).

(normal ALT levels, low or undetectable serum HBV DNA) who rarely develop cirrhosis or its complications, whereas spontaneous clearance of HBsAg gradually occurs (1% per year).[3] Approximately 20% to 30% of chronically infected patients though have *active chronic hepatitis B* (defined by elevated ALT and HBV DNA levels) and, if left untreated, progress to cirrhosis and hepatocellular carcinoma. Two major subsets of chronic hepatitis B are recognized: HBeAg positive and negative.[3,17]

3. *Past or resolved HBV infection* is defined by negative HBsAg and positive anti-HBc (total) antibodies in the serum (with or without anti-HBs antibodies).[3] Approximately 5% to 50% of rheumatic patients worldwide demonstrate this serologic profile.[18] Among these patients, a small subset (<5%) can have *occult HBV infection* defined by the presence of HBV DNA in the liver and occasionally in low levels in the serum (<200 IU/mL).[16,19] This group of patients is challenging because they can rarely develop HBVr with immunosuppression.[20,21]

PATHOGENESIS AND NATURAL COURSE OF HEPATITIS B VIRUS REACTIVATION

Hepatocyte injury during acute or chronic HBV infection manifested by ALT elevation (hepatitis) is immune mediated, as the virus does not have a direct cytopathic effect.[22] Both innate and adaptive immunity mechanisms are involved in this process,[23] including the action of antiviral type I interferons (α and β), natural killer cells, and CD8+ T lymphocytes.[22] Strong immune responses are associated with viral clearance during acute icteric hepatitis in adults, but they can also lead to severe liver injury and fibrosis during the immune active phases of chronic hepatitis B.[23]

In patients with chronic or more rarely past HBV infection, immunosuppressive therapy can lead to HBVr.[24,25] Three phases have been recognized concerning the natural course of HBVr during immunosuppressive therapy[24]: In the initial phase, immunosuppression leads to increased viral replication (high serum HBV DNA levels) due to its suppressive effect on hosts' immune responses. This risk seems to correlate with the intensity of immunosuppression and the baseline HBV DNA levels.[2] This phase can be followed in some, but not all, patients by an immune-mediated hepatic injury phase, whereby immune cells recognize and attack the HBV-infected hepatocytes. This process usually occurs after the withdrawal of immunosuppression whereby the immune system reconstitutes itself, but it can also happen during chronic therapy (as is the case in most rheumatic patients). The severity of liver damage is determined by the degree of liver inflammation as well as by the stage of the underlying chronic liver disease (no vs minimal vs severe liver fibrosis). Thus, HBVr can vary from a sub-clinical elevation of ALT levels (silent HBVr) to fulminant hepatitis with liver failure and even death.[24,25] In the last phase, resolution of liver damage occurs with normalization of HBV DNA and ALT levels.[24,25]

DEFINITION OF HEPATITIS B VIRUS REACTIVATION

Despite significant efforts, there is currently no unified consensus regarding the definition of HBVr after immunosuppression in the literature.

Most experts define HBVr by virologic terms as follows:

- An increase in serum HBV DNA levels by greater than 1 to 2 $\log_{10}$ IU/mL (if HBV DNA was detectable at baseline) or
- The detection of serum HBV DNA (>100 IU/mL, if HBV DNA was negative at baseline)[25,26]

In some patients with past (resolved) infection, this can be accompanied by the reemergence of the HBsAg (reverse seroconversion).[27] Hepatitis flares can occur during HBVr and are defined as a 3 or more times the ULN increase in ALT values or an absolute ALT of 100 IU/mL or greater.

RISK FOR HEPATITIS B VIRUS REACTIVATION ACCORDING TO ANTIRHEUMATIC TREATMENT

Here the authors present an update of the available data regarding the risk for HBVr during antirheumatic treatment without antiviral prophylaxis in patients with chronic or past HBV infection (**Box 1**).

Corticosteroids

Corticosteroids' (CS) link to HBVr has been strongly established in the literature, and it seems to be dose and time dependent. Data from several studies[28–31] and case reports[32–34] link HBVr in patients with chronic HBV infection to moderate to high doses of CS ($\geq$10 mg/d) given for a prolonged period of time ($\geq$4 weeks). In its most recent guidelines, the American Gastroenterological Association (AGA) estimates this risk to be high (>10%), whereas for patients on chronic ($\geq$4 weeks) low-dosage ($\leq$10 mg/d) CS treatment, it is regarded as moderate (1%–10%).[35] Short-term (<1 week) or intra-articular CS administration is considered a low-risk treatment (<1%).[35]

There are no data regarding the risk for CS-induced HBVr in rheumatic patients with past HBV infection. Recently, the AGA has assigned a moderate risk (1%–10%) for HBVr to patients receiving long-term moderate- to high-dosage CS (>10 mg/d for $\geq$4 weeks),[35] whereas other experts consider this to be a low-risk (<1%) group.[26]

Non-biological Antirheumatic Agents

Methotrexate

Methotrexate (MTX) is the most widely used antirheumatic agent over the last 3 decades in rheumatology. Taking into account the large number of patients that have

---

Box 1
Rheumatic patients starting immunosuppressives for whom hepatitis B virus screening is recommended

Treatment

- Corticosteroids (>4 weeks)
- Methotrexate
- Leflunomide
- Cyclophosphamide
- Biologics

High-risk patients

- Patients with high-risk sexual activity (multiple sexual partners, men who have sex with men, patients with sexually transmitted diseases)
- Sexual partners and household contacts of HBV-infected individuals
- Injectable drug users
- Hemodialysis patients
- Health care workers with exposure to patients' body fluids
- HIV-infected patients
- Patients from areas with moderate to high HBV prevalence (HBsAg positive ≥2%) and their offspring (if not vaccinated)

Abbreviation: HIV, human immunodeficiency virus.

---

received MTX, the number of MTX-induced HBVr cases in the literature has been negligible. In a recent review by Tan and colleagues,[15] only 8 such cases were identified. All but one of these patients were also receiving CS, so their effect cannot be excluded. Furthermore, in a recent retrospective cohort study of 358 Taiwanese RA patients with untreated chronic HBV infection who were taking MTX, no evidence of an increased rate of liver cirrhosis was documented, providing indirect evidence of its safety in this population.[36]

Similarly, only 5 cases of HBVr have been reported in the literature in patients with past HBV infection on chronic MTX treatment (all receiving CS at the same time).[15,37]

Altogether, these data indicate that MTX is safe in rheumatic patients with chronic or past HBV infection (low risk: <1% according to the AGA).[35] Nevertheless, caution is needed because occasionally MTX can be associated with severe or even fatal outcomes in HBV-infected patients. In a recent analysis of all adverse events reported in the Food and Drug Administration's Adverse Event Reporting System database among 92 HBV-infected patients with RA receiving antirheumatic drugs, there were 27 fatalities and in 20 of them MTX was used (4 patients with fulminant hepatitis).[38]

Other non-biologics

Although implicated in HBVr when used as combination treatment,[15,39] cases of HBVr with other non-biologics such as hydroxychloroquine, leflunomide (LEF), sulfasalazine, and azathioprine, when used as monotherapy for treating rheumatic diseases are extremely rare.[40] In a recent case-control study from Japan,[38] among 92 patients with HBVr with rheumatic disease, 12 cases of disease-modifying antirheumatic drugs

(DMARDs) other than MTX (4 hydroxychloroquine, 4 LEF, 4 sulfasalazine) were reported. Thus, these agents can be categorized as low-risk treatments too.

Mycophenolate is an immunosuppressive for which there are extremely limited data regarding its potential for HBVr. There have been only 2 cases reported in the literature[40] indicating that most likely this is a low-risk agent too.

Cyclophosphamide (CYC) is being used for the treatment of patients with severe rheumatic diseases, such as systemic lupus erythematosus, vasculitides, systemic sclerosis, and so forth, for decades (usually in combination with medium- to high-dose steroids). In a recent study that reviewed all of the available cases from the literature, Droz and colleagues[40] identified 11 cases of CYC-induced HBVr, which occurred faster than any other immunosuppressive (median time: 8 weeks).

Biological Agents

Tumor necrosis factor inhibitors

Tumor necrosis factor α (TNFα) is an important cytokine for HBV eradication from infected hepatocytes. Low TNFα levels have been associated with dampening of the cytokine cascade, impaired apoptosis and clearance of hepatocytes, and suppression of the cytotoxic CD8 I T cell responses against HBV.[11]

The association between TNF inhibitors (TNFi) use and HBVr has been well established over the last decade.[2,18] In a review of all published cases until 2011, Pérez-Alvarez and colleagues[42] reported a 64% reactivation rate among 33 HBsAg-positive patients (21 of 33) treated with TNFi without antiviral prophylaxis, whereas in 3 recent studies from East Asia the respective rate was 29% (17 of 61).[43–45] Most of the reactivations occurred a few months after starting TNFi (mean: 9.8 months); in most patients (12 of 17, 70%), they were accompanied by a hepatitis flare. Most patients (11 of 17) received antiviral therapy at the time of HBVr and had an uneventful course. Interestingly, 6 patients who exhibited HBVr (5 inactive carriers, 3 with ALT elevation) did well without any antiviral therapy.[44,45] These data clearly point to an increased risk for HBVr with TNFi in HBsAg-positive patients without antiviral prophylaxis (assigned as moderate: 1%–10% by the AGA).[35]

In patients with past HBV infection, the risk with TNFi is much lower. Lee and colleagues,[46] in a review of all published cases in the literature (n = 468), identified only 8 patients (1.7%) with HBVr. Thus, it is evident that TNFi is a low-risk therapy for this group of patients (<1%).[35]

Rituximab

Rituximab (RTX) is a B-cell–depleting monoclonal antibody increasingly used in various rheumatic diseases (RA, antineutrophil cytoplasmic autoantibody–associated vasculitides, systemic lupus erythematosus, cryoglobulinemic vasculitis, and so forth) as well as in hematologic diseases over the last 15 years.

In HBsAg-positive patients with hematologic diseases treated with RTX-containing regimens without antiviral prophylaxis, the risk of HBVr is very high (30%–60%).[27,47–50] Although there is a paucity of data for rheumatic patients (except from rare case reports),[51] one can assume that this is similarly high. Thus, RTX is considered a high-risk agent (>10%) for HBsAg-postive patients.[26,35]

RTX among all biologics also has the highest reported risk for HBVr in patients with hematologic diseases and past HBV infection. In a recent review of all published studies, Perrillo and colleagues[35] estimated a pooled HBVr rate of 16.9%. It should be noted though that in these studies, RTX was given as part of chemotherapeutic regimens including high-dose CS, which could also have contributed to this high risk. On the other hand, the respective data from rheumatic patients do not point to such an increased risk. In 4 recent prospective or retrospective studies including 190 rheumatic patients treated with RTX (either alone or in combination with DMARDs), there was only one case of HBVr with low-level HBV viremia (0.5%).[52–55] Collectively, these data indicate that the risk for HBVr is much lower in rheumatic compared with hematologic patients with past HBV infection (>10% according to the AGA).[35] Nevertheless, taking into account that definite cases of RTX-induced HBVr have been reported,[56,57] close monitoring is required (as is discussed later).

Abatacept

Abatacept (ABA) is a fusion protein that inhibits T-cell activation and has been used over the last decade for the treatment of RA. The risk for HBVr in untreated HBsAg-positive rheumatic patients has been explored in 2 retrospective studies. In the first, all 4 inactive HBV carriers who had received intravenous ABA developed HBVr at a mean time of 10 months.[58] On the contrary, none of 38 inactive HBV carriers treated with ABA for 24 months developed HBVr in a recent Italian study.[59] Although the available data are limited, the AGA categorizes ABA as a moderate-risk agent (1%–10%) for HBVr in HBsAg-positive patients.[35]

As with TNFi, the risk for HBVr in patients with past HBV infection seems to be minimal. Although rare cases of HBVr in such patients have been reported in the literature,[60,61] in 2 recent studies with 24 patients treated with ABA, no cases of HBVr were noted.[53,59] Similarly to TNFi, the AGA considers ABA to be a low-risk agent for HBVr (<1%).[35]

Tocilizumab

Tocilizumab (TCZ) is a humanized monoclonal antibody that blocks interleukin-6 (IL-6) signaling by inhibiting its receptor. It is used for the treatment of RA and the systemic form of juvenile idiopathic arthritis. Except from a single case report of an HBsAg-positive Japanese patient with RA who had received TCZ for 5 years without HBVr,[62] there are no data regarding TCZ-induced HBVr in HBsAg-positive rheumatic patients.

For patients with past HBV infection, in 2 studies with 25 patients treated with TCZ,[53,63] there were only 2 cases (8%) of transient low-level viremia that resolved without antiviral therapy.[63] Thus, there are insufficient data so far for TCZ to appropriately grade the HBVr risk in rheumatic patients with chronic HBV infection, although for past infection the risk seems to be low.

Ustekinumab

Ustekinumab (UST) is a monoclonal antibody that inhibits IL-12 and IL-23 signaling and is currently licensed for the treatment of psoriasis and psoriatic arthritis. There is limited experience with this agent in patients with chronic HBV infection. In a retrospective study from Taiwan, 7 patients with chronic HBV infection (4 inactive carriers, 3 with chronic hepatitis B) were treated with UST for 4 to 39 months without antiviral prophylaxis. Two patients (one inactive carrier and one with chronic hepatitis B) developed HBVr without associated hepatitis (at 4 and 7 months, respectively).[64]

For patients with past HBV infection, there has been a case report of HBVr in a patient with psoriasis treated with UST.[65] Although these literature data are scarce, it is the authors' opinion that UST should be categorized as having moderate risk for HBVr in chronically infected patients and as low risk for patients with past infection.

Other biologics

There have been no reports of HBVr in patients treated with secukinumab (IL-17 inhibitor) or tofacitinib (Janus kinase 1/3 inhibitor); thus, no risk assessment can be conducted for those drugs. In the latter case, one could extrapolate data from the use of other kinase inhibitors, when used in hematology. HBVr is a known complication of treatment with imatinib and nilotinib.[66–68]

Screening for hepatitis B virus infection

Since the risk of HBVr was recognized and its potential for preventability was established, the need to identify patients at risk before initiating immunosuppressive therapy became a necessity. Currently available guidelines from different medical societies propose 2 methods of screening, that is, either universal screening for all patients before any form of immunosuppressive treatment[69–71] or screening only patients who start a moderate- to high-risk immunosuppressive agent.[35]

The cost-effectiveness of such HBV screening has been scarcely studied in the literature. Screening all patients has proven to be cost-effective in lymphoma[72] (before Rituximab - Cyclophosphamide, Doxorubicin, Vincristine, Prednisolone [R-CHOP therapy]) and in early stage breast cancer[73] (before adjuvant chemotherapy). On the other hand, universal HBV screening proved economically favorable only in selected patients with solid tumors.[74] Until today, there is no similar study in rheumatic patients.

Whom to screen? Screening should be conducted for all patients who are at risk for developing HBVr during immunosuppressive therapy. Obviously all rheumatic patients who are at risk for HBV infection (see **Box 1**)[69] or with any indication of underlying liver disease (elevated ALT, any signs of chronic liver disease including ascites, varices, and so forth)[69] regardless of their treatment schedule should be screened for HBV infection.

In terms of the scheduled antirheumatic therapies, we suggest the following:

- Biologics
    Given the increased risk of serious and potentially fatal HBVr in patients treated with biologics, all rheumatic patients starting *biologics* should be screened for HBV infection.
- CS
    HBV screening is also strongly recommended for all patients scheduled for long-term (>4 weeks) treatment with CS (either with low or high doses).[35]
- Non-biological DMARDs
    ○ *MTX/LEF*: Although the available data show a negligible risk for HBVr in patients either with chronic or past HBV infection treated with MTX or LEF, the authors think that screening is required for all patients (as suggested by the American College of Rheumatology [ACR] in its 2008 guidelines),[75] because, although rare, severe cases of HBVr have been reported with these agents and the possibility of drug-induced hepatotoxicity which could complicate the clinical course of patients chronically infected with HBV still exists.
    ○ *Antimalarials, sulfasalazine, azathioprine, and calcineurin inhibitors*, have only anecdotally been associated with HBVr (usually when given with CS). HBV screening before these treatments should be individualized based on patients' risk factors for HBV infection.

How to screen? There is universal consensus among different societies[26,35,71] and experts[25,26] that screening with *HBsAg* and *anti-HBc* is required for all patients at risk for HBVr.

Whether or not to include *anti-HBs* in the screening process is still controversial.[70,76–78] For patients who have previously been vaccinated, titers of anti-HBs of

10 IU/L or greater are generally considered protective, whereas lower titers may indicate the need for booster vaccination. Also, the presence of anti-HBs in unvaccinated patients could be the only marker of past HBV infection in HBsAg-negative/anti-HBc-negative patients. Cases of HBVr have rarely been reported in these patients[79]; thus, knowledge of their status could increase vigilance during chronic therapy (especially with high-risk biologics, such as RTX). Furthermore, in patients who are triple negative and especially if they have HBV risk factors, vaccination against HBV should be performed before starting immunosuppressive therapy.[80] For all these reasons, the authors argue that anti-HBs should be included in the initial screening (**Fig. 1**) because, although it does not add a significant cost, it provides valuable information to the clinician.

The value of screening has been shown in a recent study from Spain whereby the implementation of a computerized system for ordering HBV screening tests by the physicians before biological therapy has increased the rate of screening for HBsAg from 47% to 94% and for anti-HBc from 29% to 85%, leading to the identification of 73 patients at risk for HBVr among 1076 patients screened.[81] Similarly, Droz and colleagues[40] estimated that almost 80% of HBVr could be prevented in rheumatic patients before biological treatment with appropriate serologic screening.

PREVENTION AND MANAGEMENT OF HEPATITIS B VIRUS REACTIVATION

The appropriate strategy for screening, monitoring, and management of patients on chronic immunosuppressive therapy or at risk for HBV infection is shown in **Fig. 1** and outlined later.

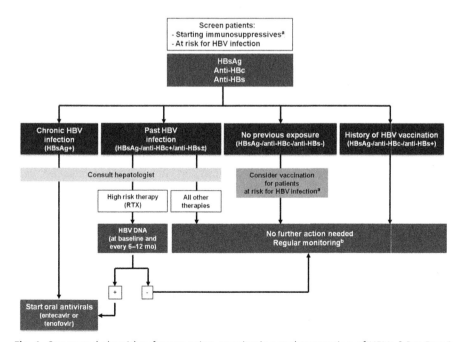

Fig. 1. Suggested algorithm for screening, monitoring and prevention of HBVr. [a] See **Box 1** for definitions. [b] As per respective guidelines for biological and non-biological agents. For patients with past HBV infection check HBV DNA levels in case of ALT elevation.

Nonexposed or Previously Vaccinated Against Hepatitis B Virus

For patients who have never been exposed to HBV (HBsAg negative/anti-HBc negative/anti-HBs negative), vaccination should be proposed, especially for those at risk for HBV infection (see **Box 1**).[80] For patients who have been vaccinated in the past (HBsAg negative/anti-HBc negative/anti-HBs positive) and have titers greater than 10 IU/mL, no further action is required. There is no consensus for those with titers less than the protective cutoff limit, although a booster vaccination might be considered for these patients.[82]

Chronically Infected Patients (HBsAg Positive/Anti-HBc Positive/Anti-HBs Negative)

Antiviral therapy for all?

HBsAg-positive patients are obviously the ones with the highest risk for HBVr during immunosuppressive therapy. The management strategy for these patients should always be designed in coordination with a hepatologist or other physician with expertise in chronic hepatitis B.

Patients with active chronic hepatitis B (defined by elevated ALT and HBV DNA levels and moderate to high necroinflammatory activity in the liver biopsy, if performed) or cirrhosis should be started on oral antiviral therapy according to the most recent guidelines, regardless of their scheduled antirheumatic therapy.[17,70,78]

For the rest of the patients, the decision for initiation of antiviral therapy should be made based mainly on the type of scheduled immunosuppressive therapy. All patients starting high-risk therapy, such as biologics, long-term CS (>4 weeks), and non-biologics like CYC, should receive concomitantly oral antivirals. There is no consensus in the literature regarding the need for antivirals for low-risk immunosuppressives, such as MTX, LEF, azathioprine, or mycophenolate, given as monotherapy. Although liver societies recommended antiviral prophylaxis for all patients on immunosuppressives,[17,70,78] recently the AGA suggested against the routine use of antivirals in this low-risk population.[83] The authors think that the decision to withhold antiviral prophylaxis should be reserved only for patients with nonadvanced liver fibrosis and when close monitoring of HBV DNA and ALT levels is available.

Several studies (mainly retrospective) have shown that oral antivirals when given in combination with biologics, including TNFi,[12,42] RTX,[52] ABA,[58,59] TCZ,[62,84,85] and UST,[86,87] efficiently prevent HBVr. In a prospective long-term study of 14 rheumatic patients treated with TNFi in combination with oral antivirals (11 with lamivudine, 2 with entecavir, and 1 with telbivudine), 2 developed viral reactivation (18%, Vassilopoulos and colleagues,[12] and unpublished data). In both cases, reactivation was due to lamivudine-resistant HBV strains that emerged during long-term treatment. Similarly, in the 3 recent Asian studies mentioned earlier, a reactivation rate of 9% (4 of 43 patients) was noted among patients on antiviral prophylaxis compared with a 29% (17 of 61) among those without prophylaxis.[43–45] All 4 patients who exhibited HBVr were receiving lamivudine (in 2 of them lamivudine-resistant strains were documented).[44]

These data, although uncontrolled, confirm controlled data from the hematology-oncology literature that have convincingly shown that oral antiviral therapy significantly decreases the risk for HBVr in HBsAg-postive patients.[25]

Prophylactic versus on-demand antiviral treatment So far there have not been any studies comparing the risk for HBVr in rheumatic patients who initiate antiviral therapy before the start of immunosuppressive treatment (prophylactic) versus at the time of HBVr (on demand).

The best evidence that prophylactic has better outcomes than on-demand antiviral treatment comes from 2 randomized controlled trials in patients with lymphoma receiving chemotherapy.[88,89] Both studies showed that the risk for HBVr was significantly lower in the prophylactic (0%–12%) compared with the on-demand (53%–56%) arm. Based on these and other observational data, most societies[70,71,78,80] and experts[25,26] recommend prophylactic antiviral therapy starting before or at the beginning of immunosuppressive therapy. Nevertheless, the AGA made no recommendations recently citing limitations of the available studies.[83]

The authors think that prophylactic oral antiviral therapy is at the moment the preferred and most convenient option for rheumatic HBsAg-positive patients receiving long-term (usually lifelong) immunosuppressive therapies.

Which oral antiviral to use? Similarly to the previous question, there are no controlled studies comparing the efficacy of the third-generation oral nucleos(t)ide analogues (NAs, entecavir, tenofovir) with the first- or second-generation ones (lamivudine, adefovir, telbivudine) in preventing HBVr in HBsAg-positive rheumatic patients. Lamivudine is a low-cost, nucleoside analogue that efficiently prevents HBVr in short-term studies.[90] However, it has the disadvantage of high resistance rates during long-term treatment ($\sim$70% at 5 years).[78] Cases of lamivudine resistance have been well documented after its long-term use in rheumatic patients too.[12,44] On the other hand, entecavir and tenofovir have the lowest long-term resistance rates (0%–1.2% at 5 years).[25] In the only randomized trial, entecavir was found to be superior to lamivudine in HBsAg-positive patients with lymphoma treated with an RTX-based regimen (HBVr rate: 6.6% vs 30% respectively).[91]

Based on these data, the most recent guidelines from different organizations[70,78,83] and experts[25,26] concur that third-generation NAs should be the first choice for patients starting immunosuppressive therapies. There have not been any trials directly comparing entecavir with tenofovir in this setting. In patients with renal dysfunction, entecavir is preferred over tenofovir.

When to start and stop oral antiviral therapy? Antiviral prophylaxis should ideally be started 1 to 2 weeks before antirheumatic treatment, especially for patients with high baseline HBV DNA.[25] However, in cases that this is not possible (life- or organ-threatening rheumatic condition), antiviral therapy can start at the same time with the immunosuppressive therapy, as it has been proposed for patients with hematologic or neoplastic diseases.[25]

Antiviral therapy should be continued for at least 6 months after the end of antirheumatic treatment (12 months for RTX). For patients with active chronic hepatitis B, the NAs should be continued until the therapeutic end point is reached as per hepatology guidelines.[17]

Past Hepatitis B Virus Infection (HBsAg Negative, Anti-HBc Positive, Anti-HBs Positive or Negative)

This patient subgroup, which comprises, depending on the geographic area, 5% to 50% of rheumatic patients, has been recently the focus of intense interest because several studies have shown an increased HBVr ($\sim$17%) in patients with hematologic diseases treated with RTX-containing regimens.[35] Based on these data and the results of a recent randomized controlled study that showed that prophylactic entecavir therapy is superior to on-demand treatment at the time of HBVr,[92] the AGA[83] and experts in the field[25,26] recommend prophylactic antiviral therapy with entecavir or tenofovir for all patients starting RTX-based therapies, regardless of baseline HBV DNA levels.[83]

On the other hand, some liver societies take a more conservative approach indicating that close monitoring of ALT and HBV DNA levels (every 1–3 months), for those with undetectable HBV DNA at baseline and initiation of antiviral therapy on demand at the time of HBVr, is an acceptable alternative option.[70,78]

As discussed earlier, from the limited available data it seems that the HBVr risk in rheumatic patients with past HBV infection is very low for CS, non-biologics and biologics, such as TNFi, ABA, TCZ, and UST. Thus, these patients should probably be handled as the nonexposed ones. The authors think that currently there are no convincing data to strongly support the need for baseline or regular HBV DNA monitoring in these patients, as it is recommended by the ACR in its most recent guidelines.[80] Obviously, these patients need close monitoring of ALT levels and measurement of HBV DNA in case of ALT elevation.

Regarding RTX-treated rheumatic patients, the available uncontrolled data from the literature point to a much lower risk for HBVr (<1%)[52–55] compared with hematologic patients. Thus, currently there is no need for prophylactic antiviral therapy for these patients. The authors recommend baseline measurement of HBV DNA before RTX treatment (see **Fig. 1**). Patients with positive HBV DNA should be treated as HBsAg-positive patients, whereas patients with undetectable HBV DNA should have regular HBV DNA measurements (every 6–12 months)[80] and start oral antiviral therapy in case of HBVr.

SUMMARY

Despite the advances in the strategies that prevent HBV transmission, a substantial portion of adult patients with rheumatic diseases show evidence of chronic or resolved HBV infection and, therefore, are at risk for HBVr during immunosuppressive therapy. Screening for HBV infection can be easily made by rheumatologists using broadly available, simple, low-cost serologic tests. Most patients with chronic infection will require prophylactic antiviral therapy with the new-generation antivirals during immunosuppressive therapy, whereas for patients with past infection, close monitoring (especially for those treated with RTX) may suffice.

REFERENCES

1. Lok AS, Ward JW, Perrillo RP, et al. Reactivation of hepatitis B during immunosuppressive therapy: potentially fatal yet preventable. Ann Intern Med 2012;156: 743–5.
2. Vassilopoulos D, Calabrese LH. Management of rheumatic disease with comorbid HBV or HCV infection. Nat Rev Rheumatol 2012;8:348–57.
3. Hadziyannis SJ, Vassilopoulos D, Hadziyannis E. The natural course of chronic hepatitis B virus infection and its management. Adv Pharmacol 2013;67:247–91.
4. Trepo C, Chan HL, Lok A. Hepatitis B virus infection. Lancet 2014;384:2053–63.
5. Dienstag JL. Hepatitis B virus infection. N Engl J Med 2008;359:1486–500.
6. Iqbal K, Klevens RM, Kainer MA, et al. Epidemiology of acute hepatitis B in the United States from population-based surveillance, 2006-2011. Clin Infect Dis 2015;61:584–92.
7. Roberts H, Kruszon-Moran D, Ly KN, et al. Prevalence of chronic hepatitis B virus (HBV) infection in U.S. households: National Health and Nutrition Examination Survey (NHANES), 1988-2012. Hepatology 2016;63:388–97.
8. Ioannou GN. Hepatitis B virus in the United States: infection, exposure, and immunity rates in a nationally representative survey. Ann Intern Med 2011;154: 319–28.

9. Molto A, Etcheto A, van der Heijde D, et al. Prevalence of comorbidities and evaluation of their screening in spondyloarthritis: results of the international cross-sectional ASAS-COMOSPA study. Ann Rheum Dis 2016;75(6):1016–23.

10. Dougados M, Soubrier M, Antunez A, et al. Prevalence of comorbidities in rheumatoid arthritis and evaluation of their monitoring: results of an international, cross-sectional study (COMORA). Ann Rheum Dis 2014;73:62–8.

11. Giardina AR, Ferraro D, Ciccia F, et al. No detection of occult HBV-DNA in patients with various rheumatic diseases treated with anti-TNF agents: a two-year prospective study. Clin Exp Rheumatol 2013;31:25–30.

12. Vassilopoulos D, Apostolopoulou A, Hadziyannis E, et al. Long-term safety of anti-TNF treatment in patients with rheumatic diseases and chronic or resolved hepatitis B virus infection. Ann Rheum Dis 2010;69:1352–5.

13. Urata Y, Uesato R, Tanaka D, et al. Prevalence of reactivation of hepatitis B virus replication in rheumatoid arthritis patients. Mod Rheumatol 2011;21:16–23.

14. Mori S. Past hepatitis B virus infection in rheumatoid arthritis patients receiving biological and/or nonbiological disease-modifying antirheumatic drugs. Mod Rheumatol 2011;21:621–7.

15. Tan J, Zhou J, Zhao P, et al. Prospective study of HBV reactivation risk in rheumatoid arthritis patients who received conventional disease-modifying antirheumatic drugs. Clin Rheumatol 2012;31:1169–75.

16. Mori S, Fujiyama S. Hepatitis B virus reactivation associated with antirheumatic therapy: risk and prophylaxis recommendations. World J Gastroenterol 2015; 21:10274–89.

17. Terrault NA, Bzowej NH, Chang KM, et al. AASLD guidelines for treatment of chronic hepatitis B. Hepatology 2016;63:261–83.

18. Koutsianas C, Thomas K, Vassilopoulos D. Prevention of HBV reactivation in patients treated with biologic agents. Expert Rev Clin Pharmacol 2016;1–11.

19. Raimondo G, Allain JP, Brunetto MR, et al. Statements from the Taormina expert meeting on occult hepatitis B virus infection. J Hepatol 2008;49:652–7.

20. Kato M, Atsumi T. Reactivation of occult hepatitis B virus infection in patients with rheumatic diseases: pathogenesis, risk assessment and prevention. Rheumatol Int 2016;36:635–41.

21. Squadrito G, Spinella R, Raimondo G. The clinical significance of occult HBV infection. Ann Gastroenterol 2014;27:15–9.

22. Phillips S, Chokshi S, Riva A, et al. CD8(+) T cell control of hepatitis B virus replication: direct comparison between cytolytic and noncytolytic functions. J Immunol 2010;184:287–95.

23. Bertoletti A, Ferrari C. Innate and adaptive immune responses in chronic hepatitis B virus infections: towards restoration of immune control of viral infection. Gut 2012;61:1754–64.

24. Hoofnagle JH. Reactivation of hepatitis B. Hepatology 2009;49:S156–65.

25. Hwang JP, Lok AS. Management of patients with hepatitis B who require immunosuppressive therapy. Nat Rev Gastroenterol Hepatol 2014;11:209–19.

26. Di Bisceglie AM, Lok AS, Martin P, et al. Recent US Food and drug administration warnings on hepatitis B reactivation with immune-suppressing and anticancer drugs: just the tip of the iceberg? Hepatology 2015;61:703–11.

27. Hsu C, Tsou HH, Lin SJ, et al. Chemotherapy-induced hepatitis B reactivation in lymphoma patients with resolved HBV infection: a prospective study. Hepatology 2014;59:2092–100.

28. Hoofnagle JH, Davis GL, Pappas SC, et al. A short course of prednisolone in chronic type B hepatitis. Report of a randomized, double-blind, placebo-controlled trial. Ann Intern Med 1986;104:12–7.

29. Perrillo RP, Schiff ER, Davis GL, et al. A randomized, controlled trial of interferon alfa-2b alone and after prednisone withdrawal for the treatment of chronic hepatitis B. The Hepatitis Interventional Therapy Group. N Engl J Med 1990;323: 295–301.

30. Cheng AL, Hsiung CA, Su IJ, et al. Steroid-free chemotherapy decreases risk of hepatitis B virus (HBV) reactivation in HBV-carriers with lymphoma. Hepatology 2003;37:1320–8.

31. Kim TW, Kim MN, Kwon JW, et al. Risk of hepatitis B virus reactivation in patients with asthma or chronic obstructive pulmonary disease treated with corticosteroids. Respirology 2010;15:1092–7.

32. Nakanishi K, Ishikawa M, Nakauchi M, et al. Antibody to hepatitis B e positive hepatitis induced by withdrawal of steroid therapy for polymyositis: response to interferon-alpha and cyclosporin A. Intern Med 1998;37:519–22.

33. Zanati SA, Locarnini SA, Dowling JP, et al. Hepatic failure due to fibrosing cholestatic hepatitis in a patient with pre-surface mutant hepatitis B virus and mixed connective tissue disease treated with prednisolone and chloroquine. J Clin Virol 2004;31:53–7.

34. Cheng J, Li JB, Sun QL, et al. Reactivation of hepatitis B virus after steroid treatment in rheumatic diseases. J Rheumatol 2011;38:181–2.

35. Perrillo RP, Gish R, Falck-Ytter YT. American Gastroenterological Association Institute technical review on prevention and treatment of hepatitis B virus reactivation during immunosuppressive drug therapy. Gastroenterology 2015;148: 221–44.

36. Tang KT, Hung WT, Chen YH, et al. Methotrexate is not associated with increased liver cirrhosis in a population-based cohort of rheumatoid arthritis patients with chronic hepatitis B. Sci Rep 2016;6:22387.

37. Laohapand C, Arromdee E, Tanwandee T. Long-term use of methotrexate does not result in hepatitis B reactivation in rheumatologic patients. Hepatol Int 2015; 9:202–8.

38. Oshima Y, Tsukamoto H, Tojo A. Association of hepatitis B with antirheumatic drugs: a case-control study. Mod Rheumatol 2013;23:694–704.

39. Mo YQ, Liang AQ, Ma JD, et al. Discontinuation of antiviral prophylaxis correlates with high prevalence of hepatitis B virus (HBV) reactivation in rheumatoid arthritis patients with HBV carrier state: a real-world clinical practice. BMC Musculoskelet Disord 2014;15:449.

40. Droz N, Gilardin L, Cacoub P, et al. Kinetic profiles and management of hepatitis B virus reactivation in patients with immune-mediated inflammatory diseases. Arthritis Care Res (Hoboken) 2013;65:1504–14.

41. Carroll MB, Forgione MA. Use of tumor necrosis factor alpha inhibitors in hepatitis B surface antigen-positive patients: a literature review and potential mechanisms of action. Clin Rheumatol 2010;29:1021–9.

42. Perez-Alvarez R, Diaz-Lagares C, Garcia-Hernandez F, et al. Hepatitis B virus (HBV) reactivation in patients receiving tumor necrosis factor (TNF)-targeted therapy: analysis of 257 cases. Medicine (Baltimore) 2011;90:359–71.

43. Lan JL, Chen YM, Hsieh TY, et al. Kinetics of viral loads and risk of hepatitis B virus reactivation in hepatitis B core antibody-positive rheumatoid arthritis patients undergoing anti-tumour necrosis factor alpha therapy. Ann Rheum Dis 2011;70:1719–25.

44. Ryu HH, Lee EY, Shin K, et al. Hepatitis B virus reactivation in rheumatoid arthritis and ankylosing spondylitis patients treated with anti-TNF alpha agents: a retrospective analysis of 49 cases. Clin Rheumatol 2012;31:931–6.

45. Ye H, Zhang XW, Mu R, et al. Anti-TNF therapy in patients with HBV infection–analysis of 87 patients with inflammatory arthritis. Clin Rheumatol 2014;33: 119–23.

46. Lee YH, Bae SC, Song GG. Hepatitis B virus (HBV) reactivation in rheumatic patients with hepatitis core antigen (HBV occult carriers) undergoing anti-tumor necrosis factor therapy. Clin Exp Rheumatol 2013;31:118–21.

47. Yeo W, Chan TC, Leung NW, et al. Hepatitis B virus reactivation in lymphoma patients with prior resolved hepatitis B undergoing anticancer therapy with or without rituximab. J Clin Oncol 2009;27:605–11.

48. Pei SN, Chen CH, Lee CM, et al. Reactivation of hepatitis B virus following rituximab-based regimens: a serious complication in both HBsAg-positive and HBsAg-negative patients. Ann Hematol 2010;89:255–62.

49. Koo YX, Tay M, Teh YE, et al. Risk of hepatitis B virus (HBV) reactivation in hepatitis B surface antigen negative/hepatitis B core antibody positive patients receiving rituximab-containing combination chemotherapy without routine antiviral prophylaxis. Ann Hematol 2011;90:1219–23.

50. Kim SJ, Hsu C, Song YQ, et al. Hepatitis B virus reactivation in B-cell lymphoma patients treated with rituximab: analysis from the Asia Lymphoma Study Group. Eur J Cancer 2013;49:3486–96.

51. Pyrpasopoulou A, Douma S, Vassiliadis T, et al. Reactivation of chronic hepatitis B virus infection following rituximab administration for rheumatoid arthritis. Rheumatol Int 2011;31:403–4.

52. Mitroulis I, Hatzara C, Kandili A, et al. Long-term safety of rituximab in patients with rheumatic diseases and chronic or resolved hepatitis B virus infection. Ann Rheum Dis 2013;72:308–10.

53. Barone M, Notarnicola A, Lopalco G, et al. Safety of long-term biologic therapy in rheumatologic patients with a previously resolved hepatitis B viral infection. Hepatology 2015;62:40–6.

54. van Vollenhoven RF, Fleischmann RM, Furst DE, et al. Long-term safety of rituximab: final report of the rheumatoid arthritis global clinical trial program over 11 years. J Rheumatol 2015;42:1761–6.

55. Varisco V, Vigano M, Batticciotto A, et al. Low risk of hepatitis B virus reactivation in HBsAg-negative/Anti-HBc-positive carriers receiving rituximab for rheumatoid arthritis: a retrospective multicenter Italian study. J Rheumatol 2016;43(5): 869–74.

56. Ghrenassia E, Mekinian A, Rouaghe S, et al. Reactivation of resolved hepatitis B during rituximab therapy for rheumatoid arthritis. Joint Bone Spine 2012;79: 100–1.

57. Salman-Monte TC, Lisbona MP, Garcia-Retortillo M, et al. Reactivation of hepatitis virus B infection in a patient with rheumatoid arthritis after treatment with rituximab. Reumatol Clin 2014;10:196–7.

58. Kim PS, Ho GY, Prete PE, et al. Safety and efficacy of abatacept in eight rheumatoid arthritis patients with chronic hepatitis B. Arthritis Care Res (Hoboken) 2012; 64:1265–8.

59. Padovan M, Filippini M, Tincani A, et al. Safety of abatacept in rheumatoid arthritis with serological evidence of past or present hepatitis B virus infection. Arthritis Care Res (Hoboken) 2016;68(6):738–43.

60. Germanidis G, Hytiroglou P, Zakalka M, et al. Reactivation of occult hepatitis B virus infection, following treatment of refractory rheumatoid arthritis with abatacept. J Hepatol 2012;56:1420–1.

61. Fanouriakis A, Vassilopoulos D, Repa A, et al. Hepatitis B reactivation following treatment with abatacept in a patient with past hepatitis B virus infection. Rheumatology (Oxford) 2014;53:195–6.

62. Nagashima T, Minota S. Long-term tocilizumab therapy in a patient with rheumatoid arthritis and chronic hepatitis B. Rheumatology (Oxford) 2008;47:1838–40.

63. Nakamura J, Nagashima T, Nagatani K, et al. Reactivation of hepatitis B virus in rheumatoid arthritis patients treated with biological disease-modifying antirheumatic drugs. Int J Rheum Dis 2016;19(5):470–5.

64. Chiu HY, Chen CH, Wu MS, et al. The safety profile of ustekinumab in the treatment of patients with psoriasis and concurrent hepatitis B or C. Br J Dermatol 2013;169:1295–303.

65. Koskinas J, Tampaki M, Doumba PP, et al. Hepatitis B virus reactivation during therapy with ustekinumab for psoriasis in a hepatitis B surface-antigen-negative anti-HBs-positive patient. Br J Dermatol 2013;168:679–80.

66. Lai GM, Yan SL, Chang CS, et al. Hepatitis B reactivation in chronic myeloid leukemia patients receiving tyrosine kinase inhibitor. World J Gastroenterol 2013;19: 1318–21.

67. Walker EJ, Simko JP, Ko AH. Hepatitis B viral reactivation secondary to imatinib treatment in a patient with gastrointestinal stromal tumor. Anticancer Res 2014; 34:3629–34.

68. Wang YD, Cui GH, Li M, et al. Hepatitis B virus reactivation in a chronic myeloid leukemia patient treated with imatinib mesylate. Chin Med J (Engl) 2012;125: 2636–7.

69. Weinbaum CM, Williams I, Mast EE, et al. Recommendations for identification and public health management of persons with chronic hepatitis B virus infection. MMWR Recomm Rep 2008;57:1–20.

70. Sarin SK, Kumar M, Lau GK, et al. Asian-Pacific clinical practice guidelines on the management of hepatitis B: a 2015 update. Hepatol Int 2016;10:1–98.

71. Lok AS, McMahon BJ. Chronic hepatitis B: update 2009. Hepatology 2009;50: 661–2.

72. Zurawska U, Hicks LK, Woo G, et al. Hepatitis B virus screening before chemotherapy for lymphoma: a cost-effectiveness analysis. J Clin Oncol 2012;30: 3167–73.

73. Wong WW, Hicks LK, Tu HA, et al. Hepatitis B virus screening before adjuvant chemotherapy in patients with early-stage breast cancer: a cost-effectiveness analysis. Breast Cancer Res Treat 2015;151:639–52.

74. Day FL, Karnon J, Rischin D. Cost-effectiveness of universal hepatitis B virus screening in patients beginning chemotherapy for solid tumors. J Clin Oncol 2011;29:3270–7.

75. Saag KG, Teng GG, Patkar NM, et al. American College of Rheumatology 2008 recommendations for the use of nonbiologic and biologic disease-modifying antirheumatic drugs in rheumatoid arthritis. Arthritis Rheum 2008;59:762–84.

76. Weinbaum CM, Mast EE, Ward JW. Recommendations for identification and public health management of persons with chronic hepatitis B virus infection. Hepatology 2009;49:S35–44.

77. Motaparthi K, Stanisic V, Van Voorhees AS, et al. From the medical board of the National Psoriasis Foundation: recommendations for screening for hepatitis B infection prior to initiating anti-tumor necrosis factor-alfa inhibitors or other

immunosuppressive agents in patients with psoriasis. J Am Acad Dermatol 2014; 70:178–86.

78. European Association for the Study of the Liver. EASL clinical practice guidelines: management of chronic hepatitis B virus infection. J Hepatol 2012;57:167–85.

79. Dervite I, Hober D, Morel P. Acute hepatitis B in a patient with antibodies to hepatitis B surface antigen who was receiving rituximab. N Engl J Med 2001;344: 68–9.

80. Singh JA, Saag KG, Bridges SL Jr, et al. 2015 American College of Rheumatology guideline for the treatment of rheumatoid arthritis. Arthritis Rheumatol 2016;68: 1–26.

81. Sampedro B, Hernandez-Lopez C, Ferrandiz JR, et al. Computerized physician order entry-based system to prevent HBV reactivation in patients treated with biologic agents: the PRESCRIB project. Hepatology 2014;60:106–13.

82. Mast EE, Weinbaum CM, Fiore AE, et al. A comprehensive immunization strategy to eliminate transmission of hepatitis B virus infection in the United States: recommendations of the Advisory Committee on Immunization Practices (ACIP) part II: immunization of adults. MMWR Recomm Rep 2006;55:1–33.

83. Reddy KR, Beavers KL, Hammond SP, et al. American Gastroenterological Association Institute guideline on the prevention and treatment of hepatitis B virus reactivation during immunosuppressive drug therapy. Gastroenterology 2015;148: 215–9.

84. Kishida D, Okuda Y, Onishi M, et al. Successful tocilizumab treatment in a patient with adult-onset Still's disease complicated by chronic active hepatitis B and amyloid A amyloidosis. Mod Rheumatol 2011;21:215–8.

85. Tsuboi H, Tsujii A, Nampei A, et al. A patient with rheumatoid arthritis treated with tocilizumab together with lamivudine prophylaxis after remission of infliximab-reactivated hepatitis B. Mod Rheumatol 2011;21:701–5.

86. Raymundo AR, Facin AP, Silva de Castro CC, et al. Safety of ustekinumab in severe psoriasis with chronic hepatitis B. Indian J Dermatol Venereol Leprol 2016; 82:326–8.

87. Steglich RB, Meneghello LP, Carvalho AV, et al. The use of ustekinumab in a patient with severe psoriasis and positive HBV serology. An Bras Dermatol 2014;89: 652–4.

88. Lau GK, Yiu HH, Fong DY, et al. Early is superior to deferred preemptive lamivudine therapy for hepatitis B patients undergoing chemotherapy. Gastroenterology 2003;125:1742–9.

89. Hsu C, Hsiung CA, Su IJ, et al. A revisit of prophylactic lamivudine for chemotherapy-associated hepatitis B reactivation in non-Hodgkin's lymphoma: a randomized trial. Hepatology 2008;47:844–53.

90. Loomba R, Rowley A, Wesley R, et al. Systematic review: the effect of preventive lamivudine on hepatitis B reactivation during chemotherapy. Ann Intern Med 2008;148:519–28.

91. Huang H, Li X, Zhu J, et al. Entecavir vs lamivudine for prevention of hepatitis B virus reactivation among patients with untreated diffuse large B-cell lymphoma receiving R-CHOP chemotherapy: a randomized clinical trial. JAMA 2014;312: 2521–30.

92. Huang YH, Hsiao LT, Hong YC, et al. Randomized controlled trial of entecavir prophylaxis for rituximab-associated hepatitis B virus reactivation in patients with lymphoma and resolved hepatitis B. J Clin Oncol 2013;31:2765–72.

Index

Rheum Dis Clin N Am 43 (2017) 151–159
http://dx.doi.org/10.1016/S0889-857X(16)30098-9
0889-857X/17

rheumatic.theclinics.com

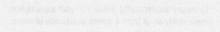

Printed and bound by CPI Group (UK) Ltd, Croydon, CR0 4YY

08/05/2025

01864696-0005